10 YEARS AFTER

PROTON THERAPY

for

PROSTATE CANCER

copyright © 2023 by Ron Nelson.
All Rights Reserved.

No part of this publication may be reproduced, stored in a retrieval system, or transmitted in any way by any means, electronic, mechanical, photocopy, recording or otherwise without the prior permission of the author, except as provided by USA copyright law.

The information in this book is provided with the understanding that the author is not engaged in rendering medical or legal professional advice. The details of each patient's circumstances are unique, so individuals should always seek the services of a competent professional.

Published by Little Pond Press
www.littlepondpress.com

ISBN: 978-0-9850823-2-1

**Dedicated To
Prostate Cancer Newbies
Everywhere**

We travel this road together.

Contents

The Game Plan 1
      Don't sue me
      A roadmap for this book
      Intentional omissions
      My readers (i.e., you)
      Q&A lightning round

My 10-Year Checkup 11
      How am I doing?
      Do I have side effects?
      Do I fear a recurrence?
      What am I doing now?
      What am I celebrating?

For Newbies Only 47
      The Newbie Trap
      The business of bias
      Risk, timing, and decisions
      Perfection and perspective
      Lights, cameras, action
      Your 9-Step Newbie-Do List

A Private Conversation with Proton Ambassadors 115
      My status as a proton ambassador
      The self-appointed ambassador
      What newbies want from ambassadors
      What ambassadors want for themselves
      Post-proton euphoria
      The impact of one

Epilogue 129

Gratitude 131

APPENDIX A: My PSA Chart 135

APPENDIX B: My 11-Year Update 139
    My health

    The Covid-19 pandemic

    Proton therapy

    Lessons learned from a dog

APPENDIX C: The Stories Behind My Books 159
    Why my first book?

    Why another book?

    The cover photos

    The humor

    A shameless request

APPENDIX D: The Best of The After Proton Blog 171
    Hank's Hypothesis: Post-Proton versus Post-Surgery

    Soup, Coffee, and Cancer Treatment

    Prostate Cancer and The Cheesecake Factory

    5 Reasons Proton Patients Are So Doggone Happy

    My Courageous Battle with Courage

About the Author 203

The Game Plan

A while ago I asked my oldest daughter on her 39th birthday how it felt to be starting her 40th year. Oops. She instantly transformed from being pretty darn happy to being pretty darn peeved. She was expecting to savor one more year in her thirties. I had carelessly robbed her of the illusion by stupidly pointing out that a birthday celebrates the *end* of a year of life. Hence, *Happy Birthday 39* means *Hello 40*. Ugh.

Unfortunately, there was no way to put that genie back in the bottle. In my defense, I have no control of and take no responsibility for the way this principle works. But I would like to point out that unlike this regrettable example in which my mouth outpaced my brain, the application of the birthday/anniversary principle can also sometimes be positive.

As a case in point, I recently had my 9-year checkup, post-proton therapy for prostate cancer. This means I am in my 10th year as a prostate cancer survivor. It gives me license to begin writing a book entitled *10 Years After*, even though my 10-year checkup is a year away. It also means I better hurry up and finish writing it within the year, before I step over the line into my 11th year.

I'm a slow writer, so wish me luck.

DON'T SUE ME

This book is about me. My cancer, my health, my life, observations, opinions, and philosophy. It includes my personal insights for newly diagnosed men—the prostate cancer "newbies"— and for the many proton ambassadors who so generously help them. Of course, you and I have a lot in common, so this book is most assuredly also about you.

Please note that I said *personal* insights. I am not a doctor, nor a certified authority on prostate cancer or proton therapy, nor a licensed psychologist. I certainly do not give medical advice (there it is, my official legal disclaimer). However, I am indeed the leading authority on me, as officially certified by the self-made license hanging on my office wall.

Just to be safe, here's a special big, bold, boxed, blatant all-caps version of my legal disclaimer for the lawyers:

> READERS OF THIS BOOK, TAKE NOTE!!!
> ## NO MEDICAL ADVICE IS GIVEN HERE.
> I AM JUST A NORMAL GUY WHO HAD PROSTATE CANCER.
> I AM A GUITAR PICKER, NOT A DOCTOR, NOR A LAWYER, AND
> I DO NOT EVEN PRETEND TO GIVE MEDICAL ADVICE,
> LEGAL ADVICE, OR GUITAR LESSONS.

Some who know me might disagree with the "normal" characterization, but what is normal, anyway? The rest of the disclaimer is absolutely true, and now it's official. However, the lack of any expectation of medical advice does beg the question: Why should *you* want to read about *me*?

Well, because I am a prostate cancer survivor who had proton therapy ten years ago.

What could possibly be more fascinating than that?

A ROADMAP FOR THIS BOOK

If there is no medical advice here, what exactly will there be? You are entitled to an early answer before you buy or read my book, and I will now tell you what you can and cannot expect to find.

Here's my plan: First I'll give you all the details of how I'm doing, possibly more than you want to know. Next, I'll tell you about "The Newbie Trap," along with fourteen indispensable insights and a slightly unconventional nine-point action plan, all specifically for prostate cancer newbies. Then I'll share my thoughts about being an effective proton ambassador, a role I have embraced and honored for a decade.

There will be several Appendixes, and because no book about prostate cancer is complete without a PSA chart, my decade-long PSA pattern is illustrated in Appendix A. Then, in case you're as curious as I hope you are, I will explain why I wrote my first book, *PROTONS versus Prostate Cancer: EXPOSED*, and why I took a second plunge with this one, which I find surprising even while it is still a work in progress. As an added bonus, in Appendix D I will share a few favorite articles I wrote for *The After Proton Blog*.

Lastly, there will be an update and an epilogue. As you and I know too well, things change quickly and unexpectedly in life. I fully expect that by the time I finish writing *10 Years After*, something notable will be different than when I first set pen to paper. I have no idea what will have changed, and at this point I have no idea what I'll say in my epilogue. When we reach the end, we will find out together.

Now let me explain what you will *not* find here, and why.

INTENTIONAL OMISSIONS

I want to be up-front and forthright about the topics I will refrain from addressing. False expectations lead to disappointment, and I want you to feel satisfied and well-served by the information I do present. If you are hoping to find information about the following subject areas, you are reading the wrong book. Or maybe you are reading the right book for the wrong reasons.

No news, no lists

I find news literally every day about exciting new techniques for diagnosing, treating, and managing prostate cancer. Some are touted as breakthroughs or potentially game-changing innovations. While I am tempted to share some of this information with you here, I remind myself that once written, my words will remain unchanged for all eternity. By its very nature, this book cannot be a source of current events because as with all books, its content is static.

A book claiming to be up to date on a rapidly evolving topic will assuredly be at least slightly out of date by the time it's published. Would you read a two-year-old People magazine to find out what's new in the life of Jennifer Lawrence?

There will be no attempt to report news or to list, review, or describe today's many medical options for treating prostate cancer. For that, you are better off carefully researching the most current information online, reading current editions of reputable magazines and journals, speaking with knowledgeable medical professionals who stay abreast of advances in their field, or reading relevant books published only within the last few months. As I said, the most recent information will never be found in any book.

If you're reading this even just a few years after publication, there might already be something newer and better for cancer treatment than any of the current options as I write. Or maybe not. But medical breakthroughs do occur, innovation will continue, and legitimate therapies generally mature and improve. Do not doubt that today's high-tech medicine will look primitive sooner than we think. With a tricorder in hand, how do you suppose Star Trek's Dr. Leonard "Bones" McCoy would view our modern medical tools?

We all continue to hope for the elusive silver bullet that kills cancer in one easy shot. Along the way to finding it, I don't expect any of today's technology, not even proton therapy, to remain on the leading edge indefinitely. Nor will Jennifer Lawrence reign eternally. But for now, both proton and Jennifer are high on my list, and depending on when you read this, they should probably be on your list, too.

No sales pitch for proton

If there is no breaking news about prostate cancer here, will there be a sales pitch for proton therapy? You might be surprised that there will not. Yes, it was the option I chose to treat my prostate cancer in 2010, and yes, I would choose it again today, ten years later, for the same reasons. And it's even better now, still on the leading edge with some very exciting advances on its near horizon.

But many years from now, who knows. As of today, we have not figured out how to eliminate cancer, nor have we figured out how to predict the future. However, I do know with 100% certainty that you are reading this book in the future of when I wrote it. If it happens to be close to the date of publication, then proton therapy should definitely be on your list of options to consider, precisely my message as a proud proton ambassador. But in another five, ten, or twenty years? I make no predictions.

Now, if you consider the previous paragraphs to be a sales pitch for proton therapy, then I stand corrected. I suppose it would be reasonable to regard my comments as an ultra-soft-sell sales pitch, and if you do, I am okay with your interpretation.

What remains after eliminating news, lists, and selling? An impassioned, detailed, candid account of my life and lessons learned throughout my first decade after proton therapy for prostate cancer, just like it says on the cover. I sincerely hope you will benefit from the personal perspective I offer, and that you will appreciate this for what it is.

And now that you know what is included and what is not, I should identify who it is for.

MY READERS (I.E., YOU)

This book is for everyone, and especially for prostate cancer newbies.

I mean, who, other than a newbie, is likely to give up even a few cups of coffee for a copy of a book about prostate cancer or proton therapy? As a coffee addict, I can appreciate that trading just one day of caffeine for *any* book would be a tough choice. If you can afford both, then you have no conflict. You can read as you sip. Or if you're in a hurry, slurp as you scan.

Your personal motive for reading about me depends on your situation, and I can think of several possibilities. First and foremost, if you are newly diagnosed you might be wondering whether proton therapy is the way to go, and a look ten years down one survivor's road should be enlightening. My post-proton decade of experience might serve as a crystal ball or a roadmap for one of many possible paths forward, maybe even yours.

I suspect that newbies will comprise the majority of my readers, and I will direct most of my remarks to them, or if you are a newbie, to you. In case you missed the dedication page, I repeat here that I have officially dedicated this book to newbies. Welcome.

Likewise, if you have just recently completed proton therapy, the same crystal ball will have a different significance because you've already embarked on this path. But I am ten years ahead and perhaps you'd like to glimpse and prepare for what might await you. We all want to know our future, don't we? Well, proton graduates, maybe—and I emphasize maybe—my present could be your future.

Or if like me, you are already a multi-year prostate cancer survivor who had proton therapy, you may wonder how my experience compares with yours. We men do this kind of thing. You know, mine is better than yours. Or faster. Or funnier. Weirder. Whatever. You might also want to fact-check me. We do that, too.

Of course, you might not be a prostate cancer or proton guy at all. Maybe you are a woman—a wife, sister, daughter, niece, aunt, grandmother, half-sister, girl next door, etc. In that case, unless you are bizarrely fond of reading cancer stories, you are most likely serving as a committed caregiver or devoted supporter for one or more men in the aforementioned groups.

After all, as I was often told by women who read my first book in lieu of their man, "Oh, he doesn't read. I do, and then I read the important parts to him." While I accept the truth of this, I'm still not sure what explains the surprising phenomenon. Maybe he's busy hunting buffalo or splitting firewood while she, as a multi-talented multitasker, is researching cancer while managing a marketing firm. Or perhaps more likely, he is flooded with the emotions of a fresh cancer diagnosis and she is helping carry some of the emotional weight by being the reader. Beats me, but good for her (and lucky him)!

There is also the possibility that you are a spy for the so-called other side. We proton radiation guys sometimes wrongly behave as though men who had surgery to remove their prostate are victims, or worse yet, our opposition. Beams versus Scalpels, Jets versus Sharks. Well, I reject this characterization. Surgery can be a legitimate option. We are not opposing factions and there is plenty of room for us all in the "I hate prostate cancer" tent. Sure, I still have my prostate, for what it's worth, and some of you don't. Big deal. The real question for all of us is: *How's that workin' for ya?* Hopefully fine.

Finally, I will flatter myself and imagine that the memorable people involved in my 2011 proton treatment might be curious about today's me. If you are one of those fantastic folks, thank you for caring, and thanks again for all you have done for me. I am thinking of the wonderful woman in the Intake Department who soothed my stress while ushering me through the entryway. And the cheerful front desk coordinator who made me and the other patients smile every day. And of course, the many RTs, those personable and highly professional radiation therapists who handled my body and mind with care and compassion at my potentially most stressful and vulnerable moments. Hey, who knows, maybe even one of my many doctors might want to read about the guy I assume was their all-time favorite patient.

So yes, this book is about me, but it's not a report on every aspect of my past decade of life. I will not tell you about my golf game (I've never played) or my sailing adventures (I am not a sailor). I'm also pretty sure you couldn't care less how well I've honed my FreeCell skill, how I've transformed my home into a smart one, or whether I prefer Keb Mo or Joe Bonamassa. I'll save those topics for a future book.

I promise to focus here on my health and the insights I've had about how we men think and feel once we've been diagnosed with prostate cancer, survive it, and move forward in life. We do change. All cancer survivors do. I've certainly changed. And life after a prostate cancer diagnosis is never the same as before. Not physically, not mentally.

I've walked the walk, so I can speak from personal experience. But equally important is what I have learned from other men and women. I have had a unique opportunity to gain insight into their lives and minds. I regularly hear from people who read my first book (*PROTONS versus Prostate Cancer: EXPOSED*), follow my blog (*The After Proton Blog*), or whom I've met when speaking publicly. What they have taught me is worth sharing, and I am happy and privileged to do so.

My thanks to all those teachers who indirectly contributed to this book, and to you who have chosen to read it.

Q&A LIGHTNING ROUND

So, what do you want to know? After a decade of being a cancer survivor I have a pretty good idea about the questions you are most likely to ask me, and I have answers for you. The details are in the pages that follow, but for those of you in a sound-bite frame of mind looking for quick and concise bottom-line answers without elaboration, here you go.

These are the FAQs, the frequently asked questions, in a lightning round format:

Q: How are you?
A: Fine, thanks. And you?

Q: If you could go back in time to 2010, would proton beam therapy still be your choice?
A: Yes.

Q: If you were diagnosed with prostate cancer today (2021), would you choose proton?
A: Most likely, yes. Depends on the details of my diagnosis. All things being equal, then yes.

Q: Did proton beam therapy cure your cancer?
A: Probably. So far, so good.

Q: Have you had any negative side effects?
A: None I can clearly blame on my therapy, but I do have some negative effects from seven decades of life.

Q: Do you think proton beam therapy is the best treatment for prostate cancer?
A: Sometimes. Maybe often. Certainly not always.

Q: Do you know any men who had a recurrence after proton therapy?
A: Yes.

Q: Do you know any men who died after proton therapy for prostate cancer?

A: Yes, but not *from* proton therapy or prostate cancer. Remember, all men do eventually die, sometimes from prostate cancer, but more often from a lot of other things.

Q: After proton therapy, could you return to your normal life?

A: Maybe, but after surviving prostate cancer it is common to see life differently and create a new improved normal, which more accurately describes the route I took.

Q: Do you promote proton therapy above all other treatments for prostate cancer?

A: No, but as a proton ambassador I do promote *awareness* of the unique benefits of proton therapy and the *consideration* of proton along with other options.

Q: Will you tell me everything I need to know about proton therapy and prostate cancer in this book?

A: Nope, not even close. Those are not the topics of this book. This book is about me.

Scattered throughout these pages you will find some useful bits of information about prostate cancer, cancer in general, and proton beam therapy, but those subjects are digressions, not the focus. The main topic is the health, life, mind, and observations of a ten-year prostate cancer survivor.

That would be me.

My 10-Year Checkup

I confess: I have not had my 10-year checkup yet, but it's just around the corner. To be totally accurate, this chapter should be called either "My Almost-10-Year Checkup," or maybe "My Upcoming 10-Year Checkup." Take your pick. I will surely reach this milestone before completing this book, and if anything has changed, I'll include the new information in a special chapter near the end of the book. Ultimately, the title on the cover will be accurate, and the information will be up to date.

In the Q&A Lightning Round I provided super-quick answers to the questions I am most often asked. Now I will revisit those and other questions, this time answering in full, glorious detail. You might sometimes feel I have given you too much information. Well maybe, but these are important questions and I do not plan to hold back. Too much is better than too little.

The questions are generally much the same, regardless of who is asking. How am I doing? Am I cured? Do I have side effects? And so on. And although the questions sound simple enough, the answers are not.

Even when the response should seemingly be a black-and-white yes or no, there is often more nuance than a short-and-sweet answer can address. On the way to the eventual answer, my brain (a self-driving model) automatically explores many side streets along the main road. I will share my complete mental roadmap with you, including some detours. So, pack some snacks and a six-pack, and enjoy the journey.

Here we go. Your questions, my answers.

HOW AM I DOING?

Fine, thanks. And you?

This automatic (and true) answer might suffice at Starbucks, but not here. In this book you rightfully expect me to tell you whether my cancer is cured, whether I have side effects from proton therapy, and how things are going in my post-proton, post-cancer life. And you shall have your answers in due course.

However, be aware that in normal circumstances, when you ask a prostate cancer survivor, "How are you doing?" you will likely get the Starbucks answer, regardless of how he is actually doing. If you really want to know, repeat the question using his name and one additional word. Ask, "Ron, how are you doing, *really*?" The last word is important, and just before you say it you should pause briefly, furrow your brow a bit, tilt your head slightly toward your shoulder, and lean forward just a little. You will almost always get a more informative response, which can serve as an icebreaker to an extended meaningful conversation.

"How are you doing" is often the first question asked of me by men exploring options for treatment of their newly diagnosed prostate cancer. For newbies, it serves both as a comfortable introduction to what they fear might be an awkward exchange, and the opening salvo of a barrage of increasingly probing and personal follow-up questions. It contains and conceals a multi-layered hidden agenda, the real agenda, with many questions within the question. And I will answer them all.

I will begin this chapter with the two big ones: Am I cured? And do I have side effects?

Am I cured?

"Am I cured" is what people often really want to know but find it awkward to ask quite so bluntly. And regardless of who is asking, the question cannot be regarded as casual small talk. Especially when responding to another prostate cancer guy, the landscape of possible replies is a minefield of wrong answers that can be misleading and even harmful, which I want to avoid.

Certainly, I want to answer truthfully. But what is the truth? It is surprisingly complicated, and it is about much more than my prostate specific antigen (PSA) history. Nevertheless, I have included my complete ten-year PSA chart in Appendix A, and I have no doubt you are all eager to see it. Some of you might even decide whether I am cured based solely on that data. So please, go ahead. Jump over to Appendix A and sneak a peek now. Then head back here for the deep dive into this tricky question.

So, am I cured?

Semantics and intent

To answer accurately, I must first consider the matter of semantics, along with intent. What exactly do you mean by "cured?" What do most people mean? I'm not sure even the person asking me always has a precise definition in mind. It seems like a reasonable question, but the asker may not have identified exactly what they hope to learn from my answer. It is sometimes a baited hook in a fishing expedition to gain any information related in any way to prostate cancer, proton therapy, or me. At other times, the questioner is seeking very specific information.

Some of you might want to know if every last prostate cancer cell in my body has been annihilated, and no one wants to know this more than I do. To many, this is the definition of "cured." No more cancer cells anywhere. Gone. Banished. Finished. Anything short of this does not justify the claim of "cured." It is a high bar, and probably impossible to prove.

If you already believe cancer is never totally eradicated, you might merely be wondering whether mine is in remission, dormant and not a present danger, but still probably lurking around somewhere. It is a slightly lower bar than total annihilation and perhaps a more reasonable definition.

You might also want to know whether I have any outward indications or evidence that cancerous cells might still be active: a rising PSA, urinary issues, etc. Some men express interest in the status of my "cure" as a means of coaxing a prediction: will my cancer ever return? Others might not especially be wondering about me, but rather whether proton beam therapy for prostate cancer "works."

Now, some men have already had a recurrence of prostate cancer. Others have subsequently encountered a different and entirely unrelated variety of cancer. Still others have experienced severe health challenges having nothing whatsoever to do with cancer. For all these men, the question of whether they were "cured" of their past conditions is all but irrelevant, and frankly, they are unlikely to ask about my status. They must conserve their limited energy to fight new battles.

I am fortunate to be relatively healthy "for a man my age." This admittedly affords me the luxury of contemplating whether I am cured of my prostate cancer. And my answer does matter, as does yours. It can affect our quality of life, as well as that of others who seek our point of view. It is certainly worth carefully exploring.

A brief medical history

To understand how I will eventually arrive at my possibly surprising answer, you will need some personal background for context. In 2010 I had no symptoms, just a steadily rising PSA (see Appendix A) that reached 5.9, at which point I had a biopsy. My Gleason score was 3+3, so I was a low-risk patient. I weighed my treatment options, chose proton therapy, and after 39 proton zaps in Jacksonville I was done with prostate cancer. YAY! Or to be more accurate, YAY-ish.

After a not uncommon and mostly meaningless post-proton PSA jump to 9.3 on the day after I finished treatment, it plunged to 2.6, 2.1, 1.3, and one year later landed at a comfortable 1.2. Not bad at all. I was admittedly envious of friends who were already zero-point-something, but I had no reason to complain. I understood that with radiation, some surviving healthy prostate cells, not cancerous ones, were probably still producing a minimal amount of PSA, which is fine. In my case, it measured a perfectly respectable 1.2.

As a side note and reminder, radiation (proton or otherwise) generally leaves some remaining healthy prostate cells unscathed. Those cells can continue to produce the prostate specific antigen, so our post-proton PSA is expected to be low, but not zero, which is fine. In contrast, surgery patients who have had their prostate entirely removed have no detectable PSA—equally fine.

All was well until the roller coaster ride began. My subsequent PSA tracking was full of ups and downs, and frankly, I've never liked roller coasters of any kind, certainly not this one.

In June 2012 my PSA popped up to 1.7, then down to 1.2, up to 1.4, and up again to 2.3 in late 2013. Yikes! Send in the antibiotics. Whew. Down to 1.3 again. Woah, hold on! Back up to 1.8, down to 1.4, up, down, up, down. Then in 2016 it hit a whopping 3.0 and we all began scratching our heads. Is it a recurrence? What should we do? How about some serious testing? Possibly salvage surgery? Maybe another round of antibiotics, just for fun?

This time we tried an alternative antibiotic, and my PSA began to behave again, falling to 1.3, 1.2, and 1.4. Then in 2018, two years after my super-scary 3.0, it dropped even further to an all-time new low of 1.0, and then to a personal record-setting 0.8!

I was finally a zero-point-something guy, not that it really matters. Well, maybe it matters a little, psychologically if not physically. It took a long seven years to hit my now apparent nadir of 0.8, but it was worth the wait. It has remained around 0.8 until the present, more than nine years post-proton. And it bears repeating that I remain a happy camper.

Except for the nerve-wracking roller coaster ride.

<u>Do I think I'm cured?</u>

And this brings us back to the key question. On one hand, I had proton beam therapy and now I have no symptoms, no notable side effects, and a zero-point-something PSA for the last few years. If there is such a thing as cancer cured with any kind of radiation, this would have to be the definition. You can't get much more cured than this.

In my situation, many men could easily, eagerly, and quite reasonably consider themselves done with cancer. Case closed. They move on with no further consideration of whether they are cured. As far as they are concerned, they are. I envy those men, but I am not one of them. Even with this stellar set of circumstances, I find it difficult to definitively declare that I am cured. Why?

For me, it's neither completely scientific (although it probably should be) nor especially complicated (though it undoubtedly is). Whether logical, subjective, accurate, or completely wrong, my 70-year-old brain has its own unique way of processing information. When I submit to it the question of whether I'm cured, here's what goes on inside my head:

The professor in my brain reminds me that all cells, including cancer cells, are tiny. Extremely tiny. Microscopic. In 2010 I had a lot of cancerous ones, and fortunately, they seemed to be localized, happily living and growing in my prostate. So we zapped them with protons and they were no longer happy or growing, and they died. Or to be more accurate, the ones that met the beam died. Probably most of them. Maybe even all of them.

But what if there were prostate cancer cells elsewhere? What if "the horse had already left the barn," as my oncologist would say? Maybe those cells did not die and are still silently trotting around aimlessly in my body, hoping to someday cause me more grief. Likely or not, I don't find this hard to imagine, but maybe my imagination is getting the better of me, hiding the happier truth of the matter.

Regardless, I cannot shake the image of these tiny little ponies of potential peril meandering around my system. For now, they have been rendered benign, but later, who knows? Fortunately, I have learned that today matters much more than tomorrow or yesterday, and I am relatively content to acknowledge the possibility of a meaningless, perhaps powerless promenade of ponies causing me no grief. One day at a time, life is good.

Still, on the outside chance these renegade horse-cells exist, maybe I am not forever free of prostate cancer. There's just no way to know without a crystal ball. But do I really need one? Truth be told, I'm not forever anything! Not forever 5' 8" (getting closer to 5' 7"), not forever clever (dad jokes are on the rise), not forever nimble (if I ever was), nor knowledgeable (once a jack of all trades, soon merely a deuce of a couple). Why should I expect to be forever free of cancer? What makes *it* so special?

It has also occurred to me that many men who have never had any reason to give prostate cancer so much as a passing thought may already have unidentified prostate cancer cells prancing around in their body, maybe even more of them than I now have, if I do have any left. After all, I've been zapped, and they haven't. So, who should be more worried? Sadly, a significant percentage of them will someday meet the monster, but I've already been there, done that, and lived to tell the tale.

Of course, I'll never forget my fear during the brush with disaster when my PSA briefly touched 3 and my oncologist offered the name of a surgeon. After that relatively short encounter with stormy weather it was all sunshine, but can lightning strike twice? I no longer expend much mental energy on this question until the week preceding each PSA test when I do wonder with more than a little trepidation whether I will revisit higher numbers.

Do you think I'm cured?

I hope you now understand my thought process and can accept my view as more of a feeling than an objective fact. And now you won't be surprised that when asked whether I'm cured, I generally answer, "probably," which is the most genuine response I can give. I have no good reason to think otherwise. I had proton therapy and by all measures, it worked.

Of course, "probably" is admittedly a bit of a wishy-washy answer, not what newly diagnosed men considering proton therapy want to hear, but it accurately reflects how I feel. At the same time, I am confident and never hesitate to point out that proton therapy was the right choice for me and is likely the best choice for many others. It is painless, precise, effective, and arguably safer than alternative treatments. It is not a silver bullet, but it's a very shiny one.

So, am I cured for good? Probably, but I can't know and it doesn't matter. Today I have food, shelter, friends, family, a strong internet connection and a good cup of coffee. I'm fine, and sufficiently cured at least for today.

In view of my now-disclosed medical history, I do wonder whether *you* think I'm cured. If you were me, would you answer with an unqualified "yes?" Or would you opt for and learn to happily live with the less gratifying, but possibly more realistic "probably?"

DO I HAVE SIDE EFFECTS?

Like the question of whether I am cured, the side effects question is trickier than you might think. I would love to simply say "yep" or "nope," but alas, my mind does not go there. Am I overthinking this? Quite possibly, but nevertheless, you asked *me*, so guess whose answer you're going to get.

Side effects are the other side of the "cured" coin. When we are treated for prostate cancer we certainly want to cure or control it, and we want to do so without side effects. Depending on your situation, one side of this coin might have more relevance than the other, but both "cure" and "side effects" are always on our minds.

For many of us, our fear of the potential side effects of any treatment is equal to if not greater than our fear of the cancer. While the disease may impact the length of our life, our quality of life is largely a matter of avoiding side effects. So we wonder, what's the use of curing our cancer if we are left with a life we imagine might not be worth living? Our overactive imaginations can be quite graphic, and the fear is real. But such a dire outcome is highly unlikely, and even if we have some side effects, they rarely reach the extremes we fear. Plus, just like cancer, they can be treated.

To be sure, *some* people will have *some* side effects, and they will treat them and somehow manage to live with them. People are resilient and we do seem to find a way to make lemonade from lemons. Thankfully, in the case of proton therapy we are far more likely to receive a basket of apples, oranges, and pears than a bucket of lemons. Nevertheless, a minority will get a lemon or two, and it is important to fully explore this issue in general, and as it applies to me.

Side effects of cancer therapy are hard to pin down because it is not always easy to distinguish between mere correlation and direct causation. As a young boy, I asked my seemingly ancient grandfather how he had managed to live so long. "Simple," he said. "Every afternoon I have a shot of whiskey and a dill pickle." He then crunched into his huge kosher dill and chased it with whatever was in his shot glass, thus presumably extending his life by a few more days or weeks. Who knows? Might be worth a try, especially if you like dill pickles or whiskey anyway. But Grampa's science is a bit shaky.

Did proton therapy result in any side effects for me? For that matter, what qualifies as a side effect? I'm still alive, and I suppose that could be considered one. On the other hand, I might still be alive even without therapy, so it's not clear whether all the credit should go to the proton beam. Regardless, assigning credit for my continued existence is not the objective of the side effects question. When a man asks about my side effects, he is probing to find out what may have gone wrong.

Before we dive into a discussion of the status of my specific side effects, let's be clear about a couple of things. First, there will never be universal agreement about the percentage likelihood of any particular side effect in a given set of circumstances. There are too many combinations of variables and an abundance of misleading or confusing data. Heck, the world cannot even agree on the seemingly simple statistic of whether one in six, seven, eight, or nine men will be diagnosed with prostate cancer. I've seen all of the above from reputable sources.

If you research the odds of any specific side effect resulting from any particular therapy, you are guaranteed to fall down a deep rabbit hole. Even assuming the available data were perfect, you will have to be more specific. What are the odds of *this* happening if *he* were to do *that*? Well, it depends.

How old is the patient? Is he diabetic? Does he have heart disease? How well does his digestive system work? What are his eating habits? Does he smoke? Does he exercise? What does his PSA chart look like? What is his Gleason Score? His staging? Good luck finding *the* answer.

Calculating the odds is somewhere between difficult and impossible. Worse yet, it is a moving target because prostate cancer treatment is constantly evolving and generally improving. I am not going to play the numbers game here. Suffice it to say, there is *some* chance of a side effect.

But what if it's you? What if you're the unlucky one who proves the risk is not zero? You have already demonstrated how you react to adversity, and you will no doubt rise to the occasion again. Thankfully, we are living in a medically sophisticated world with remedies for nearly every affliction. They may not all work perfectly, but if you experience a side effect it is unlikely that you'll be told "Sorry, Charlie, you're out of luck, so learn to live with it." More likely, you'll be given some options to address the issue. Remember, if you experience any side effects and tackle them with the same zeal you applied to fighting cancer, you can win those battles, too.

Now back to me. Answering the question about my side effects is necessarily a two-step process. First, I'll need to confess to a variety of things that are wrong with me. Then, we'll have to decide together whether any are a result of proton therapy, a consequence of prostate cancer, or neither. Sometimes it will seem obvious, but not always. Did my Grandpa truly believe he would live longer with a daily shot of whiskey and a dill pickle? Maybe he did, but I have a hunch the whiskey-pickle routine was coincidental, and unrelated to his longevity.

What follows is a complete list of my current conditions that did not exist before I had cancer and are therefore candidates for the label "side effect." It's a longer list than I'd like, but it is what it is, so please bear with me. Then we'll determine which ones could reasonably be viewed as side effects. For completeness, I will also include some alleged side effects I have fortunately not yet encountered, but others have. Luck of the draw.

I know this is a slightly offbeat approach, but it is how I view things and it works for me. Have an open mind and hopefully it will add a useful perspective to your understanding of the side effects issue.

As you survey my list of maladies, please don't conclude that I'm a mess. I don't wear any of it on my sleeve, and I'm pretty much okay. Better than okay. Awesome.

That said, here's what's wrong with me.

Eyes, ears, nose

Floaters: Let's begin with those annoying little specs of ocular debris floating around inside my eyeballs, posing as gnats, but unswattable. A few years ago, sitting with Lucy in my car in the garage, ready to go out for lunch, I found myself swatting at a gnat. Actually, several. But I kept missing them, and as they followed my focus wherever I looked I realized they were not real, but somehow *in* my eye. I figured it would clear up on its own so Lucy, the gnats, and I proceeded to lunch, then home, then to the computer, dinner, TV, and to bed. Next morning, still there. Years later, still here.

Now, are my floaters a result of proton therapy? Perhaps. I am a very different person than I was pre-proton. Since then, my view of the universe and my thinking in general has changed. Proton therapy must have affected my mind, and therefore possibly also my brain. And as you know, my brain is in close proximity to my eyes. I have to wonder whether the proton beam, maybe by vibrating my brain via my prostate, may have jarred some eyeball gunk loose. Hence, floaters.

You may be thinking this is crazy talk. Maybe so, but I can assure you I have heard a lot of loopy logic applied similarly by others numerous times. Proton therapy becomes a perpetual suspect, always in the hot seat. We automatically wonder whether it was the root cause of everything that ever happens to us, good or bad, forever after proton. And if we must, we contrive a way to make it seem plausible.

So much for my eyes, but what about my ears?

Tinnitus: About a year after proton, I carelessly (e.g., stupidly) shot a rifle from my front porch without ear protection. The unexpected reverberation within the roofed porch hit me like the battlefield explosions often depicted in movies. Instant, loud ringing in my ears. For a few days it continued and was nearly unbearable, but thankfully within a few weeks it gradually settled down to a tolerable level. These days I often don't notice it, but when I think about it (like now) I can always hear the sound of air being slowly let out of a tire in my left ear. I think it's the front tire, driver's side.

Of course, I have concluded this must be because of proton therapy. Think about it: Isn't it possible that although you can't feel or hear the beam while it's firing protons, there might be intense waves outside the range of human hearing and too subtle to feel? Maybe my exposure to two months of intense proton dog-whistling weakened my hearing mechanism in some way, making me more susceptible to damage from noise. Indeed, I was exposed to many loud noises for the sixty years prior to proton and never had anything like tinnitus happen. And then, a mere year after proton, one loud noise and kaboom! I'm a bad tire with a slow leak.

Is it fair to blame proton for this? Well, certainly. What else could it be?

Eyes, ears … but wait! There's more.

Nasal blockage: I never had a problem breathing before I was sixty, before prostate cancer, before proton therapy. Since then, my right nasal passage has become restricted, leaving my left one to do all the heavy lifting. I keep wondering what could have caused this.

My ENT says I have a slightly deviated septum and enlarged turbinates. Well fine, but that begs the question: If my septum was symmetrical and my turbinates were svelte before I was sixty, before prostate cancer, and before proton therapy, then what am I to conclude? Coincidence? Hmmm.

Again, circumstantial evidence points to proton. Who knows. Had I chosen surgery in 2010, today I might still be able to breathe in stereo.

Hip problems

Okay, you're probably thinking, "Eyes, ears, nose? Nah. Can't be related to proton therapy. Not a plausible side effect." But here is where we enter the grayer area.

How about a stiff neck, backache, or leg pain. Is there anyone over sixty who doesn't have some of this? Or over fifty? Do I hear forty? I accept that pain eventually becomes a part of life, and I would not deign to point at proton therapy for this phenomenon. But believe it or not, I know some men who have, especially when it comes to their hips.

Typically, with today's protocol (which could change at any time) the proton beam is safely aimed at the prostate through each hip on alternate days. Left hip, zap. Right hip, zap. Left, right, left, right, for a typical total of 20 to 39 zaps via the hip areas. Naturally, men with hip pain or who need hip surgery sometime after proton, maybe many years later, make the connection and wonder.

Although I know of no research into whether proton therapy causes floaters, tinnitus, or nasal blockage, the hip question has been of interest to some researchers because, well, we want to know. According to multiple sources, their conclusion is that proton therapy does not likely cause hip pain or fractures. Here are two sources:

>Whoon J. Kil, Nancy P. Mendenhall, Christopher G. Morris, R. Charles Nichols, Randal H. Henderson, William M. Mendenhall, Curtis Bryant, Christopher Williams, Zuofeng Li, Bradford S. Hoppe; Patient-reported Hip Symptoms following Treatment with Proton Therapy for Prostate Cancer. *Int J Part Ther* 1 May 2014; 1 (1): 14–21.
>doi: https://doi.org/10.14338/IJPT.13-00005.1

>"**Conclusions**: Patient-reported hip symptoms following PT for prostate cancer per the WOMAC questionnaire did not exceed the scores of the general population of males >50 years. There were no differences in hip symptoms between fraction size or number(s) of PT fields per day."

Valery R, Mendenhall NP, Nichols RC Jr, Henderson R, Morris CG, Su Z, Mendenhall WM, Williams CR, Li Z, Hoppe BS. Hip fractures and pain following proton therapy for management of prostate cancer. Acta Oncol. 2013 Apr;52(3):486-91. doi: 10.3109/0284186X.2012.762995. Epub 2013 Jan 29. PMID: 23360340.

"**Conclusion:** PT for prostate cancer did not increase hip-fractures in the first four years after PT compared to expected rates in untreated men."

Despite these exonerations, if you should need hip surgery after your proton therapy, will you wonder if it was because of proton? Come on, admit it. You know you will.

Rectal bleeding

On rare occasions I have had some extremely light rectal bleeding. Nobody likes to see blood in their stool, and I am a firm believer that blood's proper role is to flow through my veins unobserved. It should never be wasted as a temporary dye for toilet water, only to be flushed into oblivion mere moments later. But each time I see a pretty little swirl of rouge in the bowl, I wonder if it is related to radiation.

In fact, it might be.

I'll briefly explain why here, leaving the fascinating details until later in the "update" section where the topic belongs. What exactly is the topic? To introduce it, we'll need a drum roll. Introducing ...

Rectal balloons. Back in the old days (2011) when I was treated, the balloon was widely used to address the *moving target* challenge by stabilizing the constantly shifting prostate. By *used* I mean that before each and every visit to the gantry, a specialized balloon is *placed* into the rectum. Placed? Maybe *slid*? Let's go with *gently inserted.* Once parked snugly in its garage, the balloon-mobile was then filled with a saline solution to plump it up, thereby applying pressure to and stabilizing the adjacent prostate. After the zap, out comes the balloon until tomorrow. After thirty-nine of those round trips I must say, I became pretty good at it.

It worked well and is undeniably quite a clever solution. Kudos to the person who was first to think, "Hey, I know! Let's slide a balloon up the buttooskie and pump it full of a nice, refreshing, cool (i.e., not so nice, incredibly cold, and never refreshing) liquid. This will apply pressure to the prostate, keeping it still, and as a bonus the guys will love it!" Genius.

Of course, this left a small area of the rectum in contact with the prostate, which meant it could be in the path of radiation, especially if the margins around the prostate capsule need to be treated. This section of the rectal wall might later shed some tissue resulting in a little blood, typically around eighteen months after treatment. But even with this understanding, can I be certain that in my case the occasional crimson tint on my toilet paper is indeed a side effect of radiation? What about the internal hemorrhoid that's been there for I-don't-know how long? Could be that, I suppose. Probably is.

I guess I'll never know, and I'm not sure I care. I am certain nobody else cares. It's not a problem, it doesn't last, and it's extremely infrequent for me. Let's just say it makes life a little more interesting and rekindles fond memories of the ins and outs of rectal balloons.

Regardless, this will not likely be an issue for you because the old days I just described are gone, and yes, times have changed.

SPOILER ALERT: The balloon era is winding down. We men who were part of it can stand proudly together, knowing there will be few new members joining our exclusive club. Alas, today there is a newer approach that makes radiation-related rectal bleeding even more rare than with balloons. Extremely rare. For details, see my "11-Year Update" section on proton therapy near the end of this book. If you are the curious type and want to know what it feels like to the guy getting the balloon, see my Book#1 for an ultra-detailed first-hand description. It may be the only way you'll find out.

Okay, take a deep breath and grab another six-pack. It is finally time to explore the two big issues you have all been patiently waiting for. I'll bet you know what they are.

Urinary issues

No man wants to live out his golden years in diapers, no matter what euphemistic name is shown on the box. Neither do we want to achieve our daily goal of exercise steps by hustling to and from the bathroom. And we surely don't want to exchange an uninterrupted good night's sleep for hourly reassurance that our bladder is empty. If we do encounter any of these, we most certainly do not want it to hurt, adding pain and insult to injury. We just want to go when we want, with little fanfare. Is that asking too much?

Incontinence and frequency and urgency, oh my! I am fortunate to have none of the above yet. Why "yet," you ask? Well, because I hope to live for another quarter century or so, and if I do, I expect to have a pretty good shot at encountering this lions-and-tigers-and-bears of urinary dysfunction. In effect, this will be good news, the reward for achieving longevity. How's *that* for positive spin?

We both know that although I am doing well so far, two bigger questions must still be answered: Is proton therapy likely to result in urinary dysfunction of any kind? And if or when it becomes personal for me, should I blame it on proton therapy?

It makes both medical and intuitive sense that any prostate treatment could have an impact on urinary function. After all, the bladder is just above the prostate and the urethra runs right through it. You might say the prostate is sort of the grand central station for transporting urine from the bladder through the urethra and out via the penis. Is it realistic to think that radiating the prostate and maybe a little of its nearby neighbors can leave this entire urine transport system untouched?

Thankfully, the extreme precision of proton therapy helps mitigate this concern. It is notably different than conventional x-ray (photon) radiotherapy, which radiates everything in its path coming and going, including healthy tissue and nearby organs. In contrast, proton therapy delivers much less radiation on the way to the target and nothing measurable beyond it, depositing most of its energy precisely at the target, resulting in much less exposure to healthy tissue. It's not perfect yet, but it's getting closer all the time.

But prostate cancer or not, and proton therapy or not, many of us will eventually develop urinary issues, especially later in life. I expect that for one reason or another my turn will come, and I, like you, will naturally wonder about the cause. If we've been treated for prostate cancer, regardless of how or when, we cannot avoid wondering whether our treatment had something to do with it. Like others, I will feel compelled to ask myself whether proton radiation was the cause, or whether it was just part of the unavoidable slippery slope of my body failing me, bit by bit, inch by inch, year by year.

What are the statistics?

Of course, before we choose a therapy, it makes sense to consider the relative risk of urinary side effects among the many treatment options we thankfully have. But I will refrain from quoting percentages because like the prostate, those numbers are a moving target. Regardless, back in 2010 I did my best to find meaningful, accurate stats, and I'll bet you will do the same now.

Maybe, if you're lucky, by the time you read this a comprehensive definitive answer will exist, and you will have certainty about which therapy is most likely to minimize your risk of urinary complications. But determining a definitive and final answer to this question is complex and personal. The many combinations of patient demographics and general health circumstances make it hard to make a one-size-fits-all generalization. What may be the best bet for Joe might not be for you.

Plus, statistics are often difficult for a layman to accurately interpret. The nuanced impact of medians versus averages, or a possible lack of covariates might be obvious to experts, but not to us common folk. There might even be an accidental or intentional spin, leading us to the wrong interpretation. I am on the lookout for spin at least partly thanks to my college requirement to read *How to Lie With Statistics* by Darrell Huff, which has continued to be a highly illuminating best-seller for more than a half-century.

Whoa. Am I measuring my memories in centuries now?

I know you newbies are going to search for a statistically clear and conclusive answer anyway, as you should. It is certainly reasonable to want a simple answer to a seemingly simple question like, "What's the chance of incontinence from proton therapy?" And sure enough, you will find statistics, tables, graphs, and charts to shed light on this, or possibly to prove whatever someone wants to prove about proton or any therapy. Ask Darrell Huff.

The truth may be out there somewhere, but it won't be easy to find or recognize. I am not suggesting that you summarily dismiss the conclusions of others or that you ignore whatever data you may find. When taken in context along with the advice of your medical experts, it can be helpful information. But I do hope you'll also let common sense play a role. The relevant and inarguable common sense here is this: *less healthy tissue exposed to radiation = fewer problems*. You will find universal agreement about this simple concept. Ask anyone whether it is a good idea to unnecessarily radiate healthy tissue.

Who is to blame?

Someday when you and I finally start dripping, leaking, and lunging for the bathroom with some frequency, we will wonder what caused it. That's well and good, but at that point it won't matter, even if the "side effect" label legitimately applies. Because unless the cause gives us a clue for fixing or deferring the symptom, seeking to assign blame or second-guessing irrevocable past decisions will be a fruitless waste of time. And of course, having more quality time is what this entire proposition of curing cancer is all about, so don't squander yours wondering about too many what-ifs. I am doing my best not to squander mine.

By the way, you're not the only one interested in my urinary behavior. My proton alma mater in Jacksonville, the University of Florida Health Proton Therapy Institute—UF Proton, for short—has regularly asked me a ton of questions on this topic periodically since my 2011 treatment. They want to know how many times I pee in a day, how many trips to the bathroom I make each night, and how urgent it feels when I do need to go. Of course, they want and need statistics, and I would be glad to help if I could answer accurately.

But frankly, I find these questions extremely difficult to answer. How many times a day do I pee? A lot, because I'm a heavy drinker. Starting around 6am, it's continuous consumption of coffee, tea, water, Diet Coke, and if can find it, Diet Vernors, all day. I dare you to find me without a beverage within easy reach. Is it any wonder that I'm emptying all day long? Don't you? Am I that unique?

I regard this frequency as neither negative nor a side effect of proton therapy, and it is probably not a urinary dysfunction at all. Furthermore, my control is pretty good. Even when it's not urgent and I could postpone the inevitable, why wait? The bathroom is only eight steps away from my desk. Better yet, if I'm outside in our private wooded paradise with Baxter, when he empties, so do I. It's a form of bonding.

All of this is to say that if I gave UF Proton a numerically precise answer regarding frequency, it would skew their research in a way that could tragically dissuade newbies from a great therapy. My number is high enough to be misleading without context, so I dodge the question. I tell their nurse/quizmasters that I pee "about the right amount" each day, letting them supply a suitable number, whatever it may be.

Sexual functioning

I've been putting this one off because I really don't want to talk about it. It's personal and preferably private. Even as far back as the locker room in high school I was uneasy with the subject, possibly because at that age I had nothing scintillating to contribute to the conversation. Male bantering about sex is a skill I've never had. Yet here I am, about to dive into the deep end of this touchy subject. If this is TMI (too much information) please feel free to skip to the next chapter. Please, go ahead. Skip.

Here's the bottom line: I'm seventy years old and sexually active, although "active" might be a slight exaggeration and a matter of opinion and perspective. Even as I write the previous sentence, I am laughing out loud. I don't feel seventy, and the notion of a sexually active seventy-year-old still strikes me as being nearly as ridiculous as it did half a century ago when I was twenty and such a scenario was not only unimaginable, but absurd. Now I find myself wondering about eighty or ninety. What then? Surely not by any stretch of the imagination.

But I digress. Let me prepare you from the outset: although I do continue to function sexually, you won't learn anything here about the quantity or quality of my sex life, nor about technique. Sorry, this is not a tell-all tabloid or an instruction manual. I'll share information with you in this chapter on a need-to-know basis, and I'll be the judge of what you need to know. Suffice it to say, I continue to look forward to some Wonderful Wednesdays, along with an occasional Saturday Surprise. In case you were wondering.

By the way, you are not the only one interested in my sex-after-proton status [Side note: Would calling this book *Sex After Proton* have been a smart marketing move?]. My statistic-seeking friends at UF Proton have regularly asked me a few sex-related questions periodically since my 2011 treatment. They want to know if I can get an erection whenever I want, and whether I can use it successfully both with and without my wife. Well, friends, it's mostly yes. So far, so good. Mostly. Depending on how you define success.

You should also know that I use Cialis. I don't remember exactly when I started, but I do remember why. Before, during, and after my treatment in 2011 when I was sixty, I was doing well enough on my own. But messing around with the prostate is risky business, and I was aware that radiation (like all prostate therapies) can have a negative impact on sexual function. Getting older can, too, but that's a topic for another book.

Near the end of my therapy, I had a bizarre conversation about Cialis with my oncologist. I'll call him Dr. Oncomic because he is both an oncologist and a very funny guy. It's an odd combination, but it works. I called him Dr. Candor in Book#1, but now that I've known him for a decade, Oncomic is clearly a better fit. He should change it legally.

Dr. Oncomic: So Ron, you're just about done with proton. Congratulations! Would you like me to write you a prescription for Cialis?

Me: Cialis? Huh. Well, um, I don't know. I mean, will I need it?

Dr. O: I don't know, but I can give it to you, just in case (*wink wink**).

Me: Just in case? What does that mean?

Dr. O: I don't know. So, do you want it? (*wiggles his pen over the Rx pad*)

Me: Well, sure, I guess, just in case. Uh, can I try it even if I don't need it?

Dr. O: A lot of people do (*winks*, starts scribbling*).

Me: Okay, I'll save it for later. Just in case. Thanks, Doc.

***Note**: *The perceived winks may have just been meaningless blinks.*

For many months after this conversation, I carried the carefully folded medical permission slip in my wallet (just in case). Knowing it was there imbued me with a vague feeling of power. I suddenly found myself paying more attention to the Cialis ads featuring the healthiest, happiest people I've ever seen, imagining that I could be just like them. I began to wonder whether the rumors of the infamous 4-hour erection were true, and whether men so afflicted would make a glorious appearance in the ER as instructed, and if so, what the conversation would sound like at the reception desk or over the PA system. More and more often I found myself thinking about the effect Cialis could have on *me*. Although I couldn't say I needed such a drug, I was extremely curious. Wouldn't you be?

The little slip of potential magic in my wallet was burning a hole in my pocket, and curiosity ultimately got the better of me. I finally gave in and decided to give it a try. Well. I must say, that stuff really does work, and need it or not, I liked what it did for me and I still do. It's quite possible, maybe likely, that now, ten years later, I do need it. And sadly, I'll admit it's not working quite as magnificently as it once did, but then, neither am I in oh-so-many ways. But yessireebob, I still take it on Wednesdays and some Saturdays.

Want more details? I'll bet you do, like for example, are there orgasms after radiation? Well, yes, thanks for asking. Of course, there is no guarantee of this, or for that matter, of anything. But at least we know that with proton therapy no one is snip-snip-snipping around the nerve bundle surrounding the prostate while ever-so-carefully attempting to remove the organ without damaging the nerves. Those nerves are critical for erections, and an erection is useful (though not essential) for achieving an orgasm.

This is a good time to remind you that what follows is completely based on my experience, and others may have had a very different one. I have done no random *man-on-the-street* interviews on the subject, nor have I asked my proton brothers for details about their sex lives. Likewise, I assume *they* would only raise the topic with *me* if they found themselves in the high school locker room frame of mind, or if they wanted some serious man-to-man conversation about it.

Okay, enough tap dancing around the question: What about orgasms after proton? Well, what about orgasms before proton? Did you have them? If you couldn't play the violin before you had proton therapy, you probably won't be able to afterward. Not a golfer then, not a golfer now. No orgasms before, probably none after, unless prostate problems were contributing in some way to your lack of orgasms, in which case, maybe.

But as I said, orgasms after proton are a distinct possibility, and for me, a reality. But they are different than those before proton. How so? Well, assuming you've had at least one orgasm, can you describe the experience in a manner sufficiently vivid that other men could imagine what you felt? Were you even paying attention to such a degree, or just mindlessly enjoying the ride? Did you take notes? Hopefully you will appreciate the challenge I face in attempting to describe my personal post-proton orgasms for you in a meaningful way. "OMG, they are, like, amaaaaazing" will not suffice.

I know, I know, I'm still dancing. Okay, let's get to it. Orgasms after proton are different, but still pretty great, and can be equally intense. Maybe even better, at least in one respect: the whole affair is a lot less messy. While a similar if not identical sensation of pleasure occurs at climax, there is little if any ejaculate. No fluid and no squirt, although in a bizarre kind of way it still kind of feels like there is. I now understand that ejaculation and orgasm are not the same thing, and I'm happy to continue having the latter without the former. No complaints.

Beyond that, and based only on first-hand (ahem) experience, the nouveau orgasm is similar to the old one in several ways. There is a feeling of gradual loss of control and inevitability. There is a sense of intense pleasure and closeness to your partner (if any). Your heart rate and breathing rate go up and bizarre as it may sound, there is a feeling of release, even without ejaculation. All in all, it can still be OMG, like, amaaaaazing.

As I reread the above two paragraphs I realize how inadequate my description is. But it is the best I can do, and hopefully will give you at least a clue about post-proton orgasms. And in any case, yours will be different than mine, which was undoubtedly true before proton, too. My example is just that. Mine.

NOTE TO FUTURE DADS: Fertility after any prostate cancer therapy is highly unlikely, so if you are planning further procreation, you should bank some potent semen before being treated. There can still be some fluid expelled during or several minutes after climax, but it's not likely to kick any future small replicas of you through the goal posts. A good discussion of this can be found by searching The Prostate Cancer Foundation's website (www.pcf.org) for "infertility." As for me, at sixty with four terrific daughters, I decided that if I were to want a fifth it would be bourbon.

However, I would not advise using proton therapy as a method of birth control. When you research whether you can impregnate a woman after having prostate radiation or surgery, you'll find phrases like "nearly impossible" and "nearly always," but it's unlikely you'll find "absolutely impossible." Never say never.

With proton therapy, some prostate cells may remain healthy, which is why we don't expect a PSA of zero. It is also why we may still produce some amount of semen, probably clear rather than milky. But when a prostate and possibly also the seminal vesicles are radiated, any fluid they can muster is unlikely to be up to the job of fertilization. And again, the key word here is "unlikely."

Before I wrap up this chapter, it bears mentioning that the brain is intimately involved in sexual performance and gratification. It may surprise you that it is your most valuable asset in this area, and its role is critical. If it fails to perform, nothing else works, but if anything else fails you can still have a good shot at sexual gratification unless *you* get in the way of your brain (which is unfortunately easy to do).

Fortunately, as a prostate cancer patient your brain was not in the path of the proton beam, and it will have been completely spared of radiation. If permitted, it will be able to continue fulfilling its critical role in the sexual equation. So before, during, and after proton therapy, use your head and let your brain work its magic.

SUMMING IT (SEX) UP: You can absolutely have a sexual relationship after proton therapy, but it is likely to be different. How it may change is highly individual. Erections are possible, but not guaranteed. Same for orgasms. Ejaculation and fertility are unlikely. However, a view of sexual intimacy that involves nothing more than erections, ejaculation, and orgasm is a needlessly narrow one. Ask your partner what's important and I expect you'll be enlightened. If you are afraid to ask, then the impact of proton therapy on your sex life is not #1 on your list of concerns.

As a final word on this subject, I must caution you to expect your sexual function to worsen after proton therapy. Notice that I said "after" and not "because of." The longer you live, the more likely this becomes. Ah, yes. As we age everything will worsen—your posture, your teeth, your eyesight, your hearing—but not likely because of proton. When such things happen to us proton alumni, we are often tempted to blame the beam because we want to point the finger somewhere. In reality, it will be a maybe/maybe-not proposition, probably never to be resolved.

But what difference would it make anyway? At seventy, I am hyper-aware of the increasingly rapid passage of time and with it, the accompanying loss of a slew of abilities. Little by little, our bodies fail and sometimes our minds don't do so well, either (which is why I'm trying my best to write fast). The trick is to use and enjoy whatever still works for as long as possible, fighting the demons to the best of our ability as they intrude into our life.

When we find reasons to be happy and enjoy every day, we win the game of life.

And there it is. I am now a philosopher. Or am I?

Becoming a philosopher

Cancer is a wake-up call that tends to inspire us to contemplate what matters most in life. All cancer survivors may not find identical answers, but I have little doubt that we all ask similar questions. What is the meaning of life? What is truly important? How should I spend my limited time? We now have greater clarity on the importance of such things, so we continue to seek further insight while philosophically pondering life's many questions.

For many of us, including me, our perspective changes as a direct result of our experience with cancer. It might seem odd, but this is no different than any other consequence of cancer, and as such, I suppose it is reasonable to call it a side effect. But unlike the others, this one is an improvement.

What is the nature of this new perspective? I can now better appreciate that in the broad scheme of things, cancer is merely just another bump in the road. It can be a bad bump, but inevitably there will be worse. I have friends who have already hit more severe speed bumps. They have become my teachers by providing stellar examples of how to continue traveling life's treacherous roads with equanimity, despite the difficult challenges along the way. You probably know people like that, too. If you are one, I applaud you with sincere admiration.

Cancer takes many forms with varying degrees of severity. For me, it falls somewhere in the middle, neither the best nor worst bump I'll encounter. I made it safely beyond my prostate cancer and have gained a more accurate perspective of the range of life's vicissitudes. I hope and expect this will enable me to meet my inevitable next round of trouble with at least some greater acceptance and hopefully level-headedness. Equanimity.

But does our newly enlightened perspective make us philosophers? Merely contemplating life's many questions privately, confined to our own head, is not enough. A true philosopher would necessarily want to share insights with others who could benefit. If not for this characteristic, we would have never heard of Socrates, Plato, or Aristotle. We know them as philosophers not because they had deep, private thoughts, but because they shared them.

And you can see that I share my thoughts, but do I really think I am a philosopher? Nah, not so much. Plato won't have any competition from me. I suppose you could say I am some sort of prostate/proton proselytizer, hopefully not a preachy-sounding one. I just write or say what I think, and there it is.

Still, I rarely miss an opportunity to expound my musings and opinions about prostate cancer, proton therapy, and life. Whether I am an expert is debatable, but I may have more information and opinions than some others, and I'm ever eager to expound and proselytize anywhere, anytime. I have discussed the importance of early detection with my friendly UPS driver. I've explained to the owner of my favorite pizza place why a PSA test is important, even for him. These are important conversations they had not yet had.

Just as a musician is someone who makes music, and a writer is someone who writes, a philosopher is someone who philosophizes. The music may be good, or not. The writing might be worth reading, but not always. And my so-called philosophizing? You are welcome to take it or leave it, but regardless, I will continue to do it along with playing guitar and writing. I do hope you find value in at least some of it.

DO I FEAR A RECURRENCE?

Well as a matter of fact, yes, I do. Not every minute of every day, and not always to the same degree. But although I have avoided recurrence so far—or maybe to put it more accurately, recurrence has avoided me—the possibility is omnipresent. I suspect that most of us cancer survivors feel the same way, but sadly, few of us talk about it or even utter its name. Nevertheless, this beast—the elephant in the room—has a name.

Recurrence. Ugh. There, I said it.

This is an uncomfortably sensitive subject. I did my best to rationalize excluding it from this book but failed, so here we go. It's not a pleasant topic for anyone, least of all for a prostate cancer survivor like me. Or to be more precise, least of all for the other prostate cancer survivors who have already tussled with this elephant. They, not I, are the best authorities on the subject, and I have learned what I could from them. But I have had direct experience with the fear, and I can speak authoritatively about that.

Because—I'll say it again—I do fear recurrence.

The timeline of fear

As I look back on my history of fearing recurrence, I see that my relationship with recurrence has a lifelong timeline divided into six distinct eras, each with unique characteristics. In chronological order, they are (1) pre-diagnosis, (2) post-diagnosis, pre-treatment, (3) post-treatment, falling PSA, (4) PSA roller coaster, (5) alarming PSA, and (6) the aftermath beyond.

During the first era, my entire life prior to my diagnosis, this fear did not exist at all. It would have made no sense. I had not yet had my encounter with prostate cancer, and neither cancer nor recurrence were on my radar. I was probably more worried about the flu than cancer. It was a time of blissful ignorance.

Then suddenly, when I was diagnosed and became a cancer first-timer, I entered the second era, the post-diagnosis, pre-treatment era. During this period, all my fear was wrapped up in the trauma of being a newbie in uncharted territory, and recurrence was still not on my radar. For me and for most men in era #2, the fear of making the wrong decision about how to banish the cancer and avoid side effects consumed all our attention.

This short list of two concerns was all I could manage, but men with a larger radar screen and bigger brains than mine had room for a third concern in era #2: recurrence. Along with analyzing cure rates and side effect stats, these men ask, "Which therapy minimizes my chance of cancer coming back later?" They fear that even if they make a wise choice for controlling cancer and side effects today, it might prove to have been an unwise choice if ultimately their cancer were to return. They attempt to compare the odds of later recurrence for each therapy of interest. If they could find and incorporate such information into their decision-making process, I applaud them, but I could not. I had barely enough time and energy to determine an action plan based solely on cancer control and side effect likelihood.

My concerns about recurrence came later. I did not fear it before diagnosis in era #1, through completion of proton therapy in era #2, or even in era #3, the period after proton therapy, which on my timeline lasted only for about a year. And it was a good year, during which I had regular checkups, watched my PSA steadily drop as expected (see Appendix A), and generally felt relieved and victorious, exactly what I had hoped for.

Still, like most of us prostate cancer survivors, I experienced some notable PSA anxiety before each test during post-therapy era #3, but not full-blown fear. My clear expectation was to see either another PSA decline or possibly a leveling out. The latter would be the first indication of reaching my *nadir*, my personal best and future benchmark, the lowest PSA I should expect to achieve and maintain indefinitely. As long as I continued this trajectory, my fear of a reversal was minimal and manageable, isolated into brief pre-test periods. I had no concrete reason to be concerned about a recurrence.

But here is the key question: Why should I have felt anything remotely like fear at all, when everything seemed routine? As I recall, there was no discussion or mention of recurrence by anyone during my Camelot-year after proton. There was no reason to raise the issue. So why the anxiety before each PSA test? The unspoken answer is silently shared by me and all my proton brothers.

On some level, I knew that the initial treatment might have failed—relatively rare, but possible—or that despite victory in round #1, my cancer could return at any time as a biochemical recurrence (BCR) for round #2. Without these possibilities, there would be no cause for any uneasiness whatsoever surrounding PSA tests. For that matter, there might not even be a compelling reason to continue having those tests.

During the post-proton year of era #3, I gleefully watched my PSA follow the expected downward trend. I accepted my minor PSA anxiety as normal and needed no more explanation than that. Era #3 is prostate cancer's Camelot, and life is lovely. There is no reason to identify, label, or fear the elephant skulking in the background. When things are going well, recurrence anxiety is understandably mild for most of us, but whether we label it or not, it is there for all of us.

The PSA roller coaster

For many prostate cancer survivors, era #3 will continue for many years, often for the rest of their life. My Camelot period was relatively short. After only a year of steadily falling to an acceptable low of 1.2, my PSA suddenly became erratic, and thus began my era #4: the PSA roller coaster. As I described earlier, during this period my number jumped around enough to drive me more than a little crazy, and for the first time, my anxiety began morphing into something more serious. My PSA was no longer steadily falling, and worse yet, it was inching upward into the 2s. The "R" word was now privately bouncing around in my head but had not yet audibly bounced out of my mouth.

Twice during the nerve-wracking roller coaster years of era #4, I felt a sharp pit-in-the-stomach jolt of fear when my PSA hit 2.3, nearly double my prior low, drawing the attention of Dr. Oncomic each time. This was not quite to the level of a BCR, but enough for Dr. O. to show concern. Both times, on the theory that I might have a urinary infection or prostatitis, antibiotics were prescribed.

Thankfully, my PSA dropped each time. But the ups and downs continued, my anxiety remained high, and my fear of recurrence became much more pronounced prior to each PSA test. With effort, I was able to mostly put it out of my mind between tests, but for at least a week or two before each? Ugh.

In 2016 things became much worse, and I entered era #5. This tense period began when my PSA rose again, this third time to within a mere two-tenths of a point of an official BCR. For me, this was too close for comfort. For Dr. Oncomic, it was close enough to begin saying the actual word "recurrence," although it was still only considered possible, not yet definitive. Still, he was preparing me for the worst, and even offered the name of a surgeon skilled at salvage prostatectomy. This rattled me, and as a gesture of denial, I made no note of the name. Instead, I asked Dr. O. whether he was willing to consider another round of antibiotics, maybe a different one this time. He agreed, and that became the plan.

Thankfully, the alternate antibiotic did the trick, and then some. While my fear remained steady, my PSA swiftly dropped from 3.0 all the way back to 1.3, and then 1.2. I was able to breathe again, feeling that I had dodged a bullet. But the next reading was 1.4, to which I reacted with an internal, "Oh, no. Here we go again." As you can imagine, even though 1.4 was technically fine, I was not.

Although I did not know it at the time, my era #5 was ending. This notorious period which began at a PSA of 3.0 and continued for two years, was finally winding down, transitioning into the next segment on my timeline, the one in which the magic happened.

The unexpected magic

After my PSA popped to 1.4 again, it quickly dropped unexpectedly to 1.0. This totally unanticipated milestone was the lowest it had been—ever! My emotions were extreme and mixed. Of course, given my flirtation with BCR, I was relieved, while also excited and just plain happy. At the same time, I could not help but feel it was a mistake, and it would be prudent to prepare for disappointment next time. After all, this was seven years after proton, a long time to reach a nadir. Hope for the best, expect the worst, remain vigilant. Beware the beast.

Even as era #6 began, I could initially only feel reserved optimism rather than confidence. My fear of recurrence was still bonafide fear and had not yet reverted to the milder anxiety of earlier eras. I had already learned that my PSA could be a fickle fellow, so being disappointed again would come as no surprise. I could easily imagine a PSA of 1.7 six months later. But at least I was able to again confine most of my fear to the few days immediately preceding each test. I wanted to enjoy it while I could.

And then, magically, it fell again, this time to ... wait for it ... wait for it ... 0.8. Yes, that's right. ZEEEERO POINT eight! Another new lifetime low, where it has remained for three years so far, tapping 0.9 only twice. And now, strange as it feels, I would be more surprised to see a higher PSA than another 0.8 or 0.9. With a stable, low PSA throughout the most recent years of my post-proton decade, I can finally relax for the first time since my roller coaster began.

I am still in my magical era #6 but make no mistake about it: The elephant is still in my room. Even though I now have good evidence that it has lost interest in me, it has not left the room. Only Elvis has left the room.

The path forward

None of us want to go a second round with prostate cancer, but if we do, we can tackle it. Just like the first time. In round #1 we discovered the amazing option of proton therapy to treat our cancer. Likewise, we will find an ever-increasing number of new, creative, and effective methods of diagnosing and treating a recurrence, if necessary.

With proton therapy we are unlikely to have debilitating side effects or a second battle with prostate cancer, but we might. And every possible outcome is one of many side streets of the main road we travel together. When one of us finds himself in uncharted territory, the rest of us will be there to support him and if asked, help navigate.

The men I know who have had a recurrence often react first with a slow, deep breath of anticipated exhaustion, followed by a dejected, "Why me?" Then they hunker down and get to work. The specifics of their situations vary greatly, and the path forward is equally varied. But there is a path forward for each of them, and if you or I must face recurrence, we will find our paths, too.

Those of us who fortunately do not have to ask "why me" often nevertheless wonder "what if me." I mention this again to emphasize the importance of remembering that we are all in the same boat of uncertainty regarding our future, and we need to stick together. The bond I share with all my proton brothers is not broken because of recurrence. Neither theirs nor mine.

Sadly, I have seen men who experience recurrence withdraw from the rest of us, isolating themselves from our support precisely when they need it most. There are many understandable reasons for this, but a self-imposed exile is unfortunate and unnecessary. If you have a recurrence, I am here for you and want to help. Our shared past remains intact, and I am well-aware that your unexpected future could become mine. We both remain in the same large boat, and you have not become a man overboard.

People who have not had a bout with the big "C" may believe that once we cancer survivors have "cured" our cancer, we are done with it. While we certainly wish this were true, we have seen the elephant. Life after cancer is never the same, and for cancer survivors, the possibility and perhaps also fear of a recurrence, unlikely as it may be, is forever part of it.

But we can live with it. And we can appreciate the days between PSA tests even more than we might have without having made the journey. Our enhanced awareness of our precious, limited time is the reason we cancer survivors often ironically claim to be lucky to have had the awakening that cancer provided.

My life is better, and I am arguably a better person because of a bit of bad news along the way.

WHAT AM I DOING NOW?

I have seen a plethora of proton therapy patient testimonials including articles and videos. They are touching and inspiring. They depict vibrant men who have fought the good fight and returned to a normal, active life of boating, fishing, golfing, parasailing, bungee-jumping, hiking, mountain climbing, horseback riding, scuba diving, professional wrestling, and race car driving.

You'll no doubt be thrilled to know that a decade after my prostate cancer and proton therapy, I too am continuing all my usual activities, although the intensity of my imagery might not match that of those other amazing survivors. I continue to not play golf, not play tennis, not run marathons, not parasail, not free solo, not scuba dive, and not care about or watch football, baseball, or basketball on TV. Also, I remain a big fan of not traveling, although someday my reluctance to venture farther from home than my favorite local pizza place might lessen a little.

I do play my guitars, explore and experiment with technology, and use my elliptical for an hour most days while watching tennis on TV. Baxter still takes me on our daily walk in the woods, although he's 16 years old and our walks are less frequent and less vigorous. And as you can see, my writing continues. Slowly. Plugging away at my computer, composing articles for *The After Proton Blog* and other writing projects which may or may not come to fruition. Someday I might even write about something totally unrelated to prostate cancer or proton therapy, if there is such a thing.

In the world of prostate cancer and proton therapy, I am more involved than I would have ever imagined. Maybe more active than most, yet much less so than many laudable leaders who have had a huge influence. Their efforts impact the lives of thousands of prostate cancer patients. For me, it is more of a one-by-one effort.

My name and number remain on the ambassador list for the University of Florida Health Proton Therapy Institute, my proton alma mater. Hopefully, each person who called me found our conversation to be worthwhile. Those discussions have certainly been time well spent for me, and I will always be willing to take time to talk with newbies. As they hope to learn something useful from me, I invariably gain insight from them.

I still do occasional public speaking on prostate cancer and proton therapy, and also expect to continue writing on those topics, as time permits. Some scintillating new articles are likely to join the many dozens already posted for free on *The After Proton Blog*. And guess what: I'm writing another book (this one). Once it is finished, some back-burnered music and technology projects, my version of a bucket list, may finally be able to move back to the front burner.

Most importantly, I endeavor to be the best husband and ceramics studio assistant I can be for my wife Lucy, the love of my life. This means supporting her pursuits, far more interesting than mine, and tackling as much as possible from the honey-do list which she updates continually, outpacing my ability to keep up. But brownie points are the currency of life, and I accumulate as many as I possibly can.

So, what are *you* doing? How many brownie points have you earned today?

WHAT AM I CELEBRATING?

I have a good life. I am thankful for it every day, and constantly aware of winning life's lottery, living in a beautiful slice of heaven in rural South Carolina with the woman of my dreams. My four daughters are married, happy, healthy, and self-sufficient. My eight grandkids are a delight. My 97-year-old mother is still enjoying a life many 80-year-olds would envy. I have a few good friends, a loyal canine companion, and time in retirement to do things like write books.

However, as you may know, I had cancer. Ironically, I can also celebrate the opportunity cancer has given me to help others. I've never been much of a do-gooder, opting instead for a rather reclusive and sadly self-centered lifestyle. But as a cancer survivor and proton ambassador I've learned how to (pardon the trite phrase) give back, which is definitely worth celebrating. Suffice it to say that cancer has made me a better person. Go figure.

Last May I celebrated my seventieth birthday. I am now saddled with the official designation of "old man," and not feeling especially celebratory about the label. But you won't hear me say I'm seventy-years young, a dead giveaway that I'm not. Nor will I claim that seventy is the new fifty. I'm seventy, not fifty. I knew people who did not make it to seventy, so I am especially happy and eager to celebrate that I somehow did.

Who knows, without proton therapy over nine years ago I might not have made it to seventy, and I have been celebrating that life-changing event for nearly a decade, some of the most gratifying years of my life. The book you are now reading is my effort to share this experience with you. And you *are* reading it, which means I have at least one reader, so thanks for giving me another reason to celebrate!

And then there's Lucy. I celebrate my good fortune of finding her, and that she married me over a quarter century ago despite a boatload of baggage I carried at the time. It remains a mystery to me why she hopped onto this fast-moving train when she did, but the fact that she has stuck around, still loves me, and lets me love her is something I celebrate every minute of every day.

Oops. I almost forgot. There's one more thing to celebrate.

No. More. Prostate. Cancer.

* * * * *

That's enough about me. Now, what about you? How are *you* doing? Are you also a decade post-treatment?

Or are you a newbie? Yes? Then read on. The next section is especially for you.

For Newbies Only

I have already used the term numerous times in previous chapters, and now I am officially asking: Are you a *newbie*? More specifically, are you a *prostate cancer* newbie? Probably. After all, you chose to read this book rather than a scintillating spy thriller. You may also be a *proton* newbie. If you are either or both, then you are in precisely the right place. This chapter is specifically for you, although trespassers are also welcome.

If you skipped the previous chapters and jumped directly here, you are unaware that I lied a little at the outset. I said this book is strictly about me. Well, I must now modify my earlier statement because although this chapter is certainly coming from inside my head, it is most definitely about you. That is, if you are just getting your feet wet with prostate cancer, proton therapy, or both.

Yep. You are a newbie.

And you're in luck because I happen to know a lot about prostate cancer newbies. I have spoken with hundreds, I once was one, and as they say, it takes one to know one. So let me be blunt. Newbies do not always think as clearly as they did pre-cancer. The whole world suddenly seems different, and the future can understandably look a little cloudy. Cancer tends to have that effect on mere mortals like us.

My initial mindset as a newbie was simple: My overriding objective was to clear the fog and find the road back to my pre-cancer "normal" life ASAP. A newbie's focus is to survive and then thrive. Killing the cancer feels urgent, like quickly stomping on a fast-moving spider. Still, a newbie does not want to make any hasty decisions, so he tries to slow down as he speeds up. Which would be a neat feat if he could pull it off, but the effort probably leaves him exhausted and tied up in psychological knots.

This is not the best mindset for making a life-changing, no-do-over kind of decision like choosing a prostate cancer therapy. Key concepts that are clear in calmer times suddenly become fuzzy or forgotten. Facts of life that are normally obvious may seem more obscure. Clear-minded decision-making mechanisms just don't work when a man-eating monster is hot on your trail.

I remember it well, and I'd like to help.

Here's what I can do: I will explore some crucial concepts to keep in mind as you chart your course. You may or may not already know these, but as I said, you might not be thinking as clearly as you usually do, and some reminders certainly can't hurt. But please do keep in mind that I am not a doctor (sorry, Mom) and cannot pretend to know what you should do, medically speaking. Nevertheless, I can and will share a decade's worth of memories, insights, and observations that can help you navigate to a good decision.

Navigate? Chart your course? Sounds like some kind of a road trip. I'm sure you have noticed, as have I, that many people do refer to this bizarre period as a journey, and it is. But it's more than that. On an everyday sort of journey you simply roll down your windows, set your cruise control to a safe speed (or engage the auto-drive feature if available), and happily cruise from one place to another enjoying the breeze and the scenery along the way.

This journey will be different.

Just as the *prostate cancer club* is one that nobody chooses to join, the journey faced by a newbie is an *adventure* nobody wants to go on. There will be challenges, obstacles, rewards, decisions, the unknown, and the unexpected, just like a good Stephen King novel or a Parker Brothers board game. The goal is to safely arrive at the desired destination, and because the outcome will feel uncertain, the suspense will be heightened. Are you beginning to get excited? Can you feel the thrill?

If you pay attention along the way, you will be rewarded with at least a few fantastic stories to share later in life. This is one of the bonuses of having prostate cancer, so take detailed notes. I can assure you that your friends and family of all generations will be a captive audience, excited and eager to hear again and again and again and again how you conquered prostate cancer. You should start practicing now, even before the story is complete.

You will find a lot of detail in this section "For Newbies Only," so grab a beer and some peanuts and settle into a comfortable chair.

Prepare to take a deep dive into the topics of bias, risk, timing, decision-making, perfection, and perspective—critical components of your newbie adventure. Then, once you have digested all this (including the beer and peanuts), I will provide an action plan in the next section, "Your 9-Step Newbie-Do List."

If you are a fast reader you can warm up your Chevy now, but don't put it in gear yet. Sit tight until I tell you about one of the major potholes you'll encounter on the road ahead.

THE NEWBIE TRAP

Our natural hunger for hope as a newbie leads us to a trap, one you could fall into even while reading this book. The trap is not obvious, but common and seductive. That's why it's a trap. So, to help you avoid this dangerous pitfall/pothole even now while reading this book, I have promoted it to the top of the Newbies chapter.

As much as I'd like to just give you the bottom line—the trap—you will need some background for it to make sense. And while I paint the picture, please have some patience because I paint slowly, with a lot of detail. When I eventually define the trap, you might say, "Aha, I already knew that!" If so, pat yourself on the back (if your rotator cuff cooperates). You're already ahead of more than a few others.

To facilitate our discussion, let's consider a hypothetical prostate cancer newbie. Even a fictitious man needs a good name, so should we call him Newb? Or Newt? Or Ewbie? I like Newt. Let's go with that. But if you are a prostate cancer newbie, maybe we don't need a fictitious guy at all, in which case you can find-and-replace "Newt" with your own name. You would use Ctrl+H on some systems.

Let's start by taking a close look at a key component of Newt's due diligence.

Contacting past patients

Having just learned he has prostate cancer, Newt is doing all he can to figure out the right approach to deal with it. He wants to be thorough, and as is the case with many if not most newbies, his research includes contacting other prostate cancer survivors. To many of us, such conversations feel like the most important part of our due diligence. It certainly felt that way to me in 2010 when I spent two hours with a local proton graduate (thanks, Harold) over a cup of coffee at Barnes and Noble, picking his brain until there was little left of it.

I would not have even considered proton or any other therapy without first talking with past patients. Heck, I won't even try a new burger joint without checking the 5-star rating and reading what past patrons have to say. Why should I waste my limited time or money on a sub-standard sandwich or sloppy service? I need to know in advance exactly what to expect, and with information as readily available as it is now, I can find out, so I do. Indeed, I must!

It's the same general idea when it comes to cancer, but a 5-star system will not suffice. Newt wants to read patient testimonials, and even more importantly, he wants to have at least a few two-way conversations. For some therapies it is not easy or even possible to find a list of past patients willing to talk, but Newt is pleased to discover that with proton therapy there is often a list of volunteers, ambassadors like me who have given permission to their treatment facility to share their contact information with newbies. They, or rather, *we* are very willing to speak with Newt, as others once spoke with us.

Newt may see dozens or even hundreds of names on a proton ambassador list, which is reassuring in and of itself. As much as he would like to, he cannot call them all, so he looks for men his age who live near him, or he may look for men treated many years ago (like me) to see if they're still kicking (like me). He will be methodical, keeping careful notes in a spiral notebook, or if he is a fellow computer nerd, in a spreadsheet. Because for Newt, contacting us seems like an especially crucial part of his decision-making process.

But is it? And more importantly, should it be?

Well, yes, absolutely, if Newt can avoid the trap.

This begs the question I have often asked myself when my phone rings: why did Newt really contact me? What does he realistically expect to learn by talking with me or any other proton alumnus? Does he even know? Exactly why does it feel like such an essential part of his due diligence?

On the surface it certainly seems like an obvious and potentially valuable thing to do, and in most respects, except for one which is the trap, it is. Doing so helps us feel less alone and gives us hope that our cancer can be controlled while affording us good quality of life, exactly the picture we want to paint. Talking with a satisfied survivor who has been there, done that, and understands our plight provides this kind of reassurance.

There is also the matter of trust. Newt is confident that other men who have walked in his shoes will shoot straight with him. He may be less confident, and perhaps rightfully so, that some medical professionals and treatment facilities will be as unbiased as a fellow prostate cancer survivor (more on this later). Nor does he expect them to understand or appreciate how he truly feels unless they have coincidentally also walked the walk.

Newt is naturally more comfortable asking other men in his boat about the sensitive matters he must now confront. He is feeling a bit alone, and he is looking for a brotherly kinship with trustworthy men who "get it." Fortunately, we ambassadors are highly qualified in this regard. Of course, Newt also wants reliable information and as a potential bonus, some guidance, and we do remarkably well in those areas, too. When we speak to Newt, he listens carefully,

When we survivors are contacted, we are instantly empowered to provide support, information, and direction that Newt will take to heart. In our conversations with him we can provide invaluable and trustworthy reassurance, encouragement, and empathy. But there is one thing we cannot offer, something Newt might mistakenly infer, maybe even subconsciously.

Twisted statistics

Now, I realize that despite my inevitable future status as a world-famous best-selling author, I am unlikely to be the only one Newt calls. He instinctively knows that a sample of one is not sufficient. One man's story, even one as scintillating as mine, is just one story. So, Newt calls some others to be sure he is getting the big picture. The *full* picture. But how many are enough? He will continue calling proton graduates until he either detects a consensus or feels there is no new information to be obtained, and for Newt, that will be enough.

Let's suppose Newt calls twenty proton alumni, which is probably on the high side for most of us. He will gather a lot of information and it would all seem relevant and very important, but Newt also wants to be sure it is valid. He therefore needs to feel confident he has contacted *plenty* of guys, enough to corroborate what he has heard and justify the conclusion he has reached.

But unfortunately, twenty is not much more statistically significant than one. While it might be obvious to Newt that talking with just one man is not enough, he may feel that twenty is, well, plenty. And in some ways, it is, but not statistically. Whether twenty or fifty, and whether they all agree or have mixed opinions and experiences, Newt will not have conducted a scientifically randomized study of prostate cancer survivors who had proton therapy. He will have heard a few interesting anecdotal stories, and that is all.

Admittedly, the most emotionally compelling stories you will ever hear are from men who have already been treated for prostate cancer, and from their wives, children, and others who know them. Whether happy or sad, those stories will be detailed, personal, and heartfelt. You will detect a hidden plea to *please do this, too*, or occasionally *please avoid this if you can*. Your natural reaction justifiably will be either *I would sure like the same outcome as his*, or maybe *I definitely don't want that to happen to me*.

Before you start making calls, open your math book, the one you kept (and cherish) from your favorite class. Turn to the chapter on probability and ask yourself this (be careful; it's a trick question): If you speak with as many as ten surgery patients, three of whom are at least somewhat unhappy, does that mean that surgery has a thirty percent chance of unsatisfactory results? If you speak with ten radiation patients and they are all thrilled with and enthusiastic about their experience, can you conclude that radiation is 100% perfect? Neither conclusion is justified, as you will undoubtedly agree now, while in your most analytical frame of mind. But later, with a bear in hot pursuit, you may feel a compelling temptation to draw unscientific conclusions as you listen to these impassioned patient stories.

Hopefully Newt will have read this book and will be on the alert for the scenario I just described. He will then know, and hopefully remember, that although such inspiring stories can be highly inspiring and influential, they are not statistically meaningful. But they can be so compelling—we ambassadors are excellent storytellers—that only with a conscious effort will you or Newt be able to resist the temptation to make a decision based on a few *statistically* insignificant subjective stories. *It worked for Joe, so it should work for me* does not represent sound judgment. Neither does *it was a disaster for Joe, so I better not do what he did* represent good thinking. The statistically worst treatment available can have some successes. The statistically best treatment available can have some poor outcomes, too.

BUT—and here is where it gets tricky—even if you know that basing your decision on the few random stories you happen to hear is not a scientifically valid approach, might it be reasonable to do so, anyway?

Yep.

I can hear you saying, "Wow, Ron. You just spent many paragraphs convincing me not to put much stock into the patient stories I hear, and now you are saying it's okay to base my decision on those stories. Well, Ron, old buddy. Which is it? Make up your mind!"

Okay, let me explain. The crux of the matter is that the decision-making mechanism that works best for Newt might not be the same as the one that works for you or me. We each go about our lives with our own unique approach to the choices we must make. Some of us dig wide and deep, looking for even the most obscure tidbits of data that might be even remotely relevant to the matter at hand. Others just look for a warm vibe and then follow their gut. Who am I to say which approach is better for Newt? Science is not for everyone all the time, and that's okay.

Where does that leave us, other than confused? Where does it lead?

Aha. At last, it leads us to The Newbie Trap.

The Newbie Trap, revealed

What exactly is The Newbie Trap? By now you can probably define it yourself, but here is my definition:

> **The Newbie Trap is** a newbie's natural inclination to attribute supreme significance to input from just a few past patients. When he accepts these anecdotal stories as statistically meaningful and then makes his treatment decision based on this highly seductive part of his research, he has fallen into the trap.

It is fine to follow your patient-inspired instincts as long as you do so with eyes wide open, seeing and accepting that it is not a scientifically valid approach. If you are willing to purposefully do this, then you are in the clear. It would make you one of many people who trust their feelings without necessarily needing validation from the math and science community. If that's you, your life is enviably much simpler than mine because I am on the opposite end of the spectrum, very likely overthinking a lot of things.

For you, this is not a trap because it is a conscious recognition of how you prefer to address this challenge.

But you do have to own it. If you delude yourself into believing that your conversations are more than anecdotal, you are mistaken. If you cannot be honest with yourself now, then you may easily fall into the trap and later regret your decision and the flawed process that led you to it.

I often hear newbies begin a description of their experience contacting past patients in similar ways. "I talked with a bunch of guys and they all …" Or maybe, "I spoke with about a dozen proton patients and without exception …" Or perhaps, "Wow, I couldn't find *any* proton men who ..." Or possibly, "It's amazing! Only one guy had a minor issue with ..." All of these remarks are evidence that The Newbie Trap is in play.

When a newbie says, "I've spoken with fifteen men and every single one of them is a happy camper, so it looks like proton therapy is *logically* the way to go," he has fallen head-first into The Newbie Trap. If he were to somehow find a dozen unhappy proton men and concluded that proton is to be avoided, he would still have been trapped. Or fifty-fifty, happy-unhappy, so proton is clearly iffy? Trapped again.

Past patients, especially ambassadors, are uniquely able to provide reassurance, empathy, and help with navigating the journey you are on. And you can greatly benefit from their experience while remaining mindful of the trap. Even as you read this book, please remember that it is merely about me, and I am but one data point: an unscreened, self-appointed ambassador, and not a medical expert. I have done well with proton therapy, and I encourage you to consider it, too.

If this is sufficient for you and you feel no need to dig further, then I, along with any other ambassadors you have contacted, am happy to have empowered you to confidently forge ahead with proton therapy. Just go for it and don't look back. But I hope you do so also, at least in part, because you understand proton's unique characteristics as compared with other treatments, not merely because I did so well (trapped?) or because I speak convincingly with great passion (trapped?).

If you would like me to show you some cool guitar licks, I can, and you don't need to validate what you learn with any other source. If you are hungry for some spreadsheet tricks, I'm your man. As a retired IT guy I know a bunch, and you need look no further. And if you want to know a good way to deal with prostate cancer, I can tell you about my experience, but it is up to you to be wary of The Newbie Trap.

Before you move bravely ahead, read the above definition several times, think about it carefully, and digest it fully. Do your best to avoid falling into The Newbie Trap, and while you're at it, remember to also watch out for some other inevitable bumps on this rocky road, bumps that are not always easy to spot, bumps that are commonly labeled with this common 4-letter word, worthy of another drum roll:

B-I-A-S. Ugh.

THE BUSINESS OF BIAS

Bias is a 4-letter word with a negative connotation. Plain and simple, bias is bad, right? In my twisted brain, bias overlaps bigotry and prejudice in a messy Venn diagram that might not necessarily be an accurate representation of the truth.

We do need the truth about bias because it is unavoidable, and it's everywhere. This is relevant to you now because on your exciting prostate cancer adventure you will have to identify it, evaluate it, and deal with it. But you will not have to wonder case-by-case if so-and-so has a bias. The answer is yes. Every time. Count on it.

If you are a gut-instinct style quick decision maker, none of this chapter will matter to you. But if you are a researcher (well of course you are, you're reading books about prostate cancer) you will soon find yourself sifting through mountains of information and advice about how to deal with it. With rare exception, your friends, family, medical experts, public speakers, and authors (ahem) will all have input for you.

And they are all biased. Even you are biased, and so am I.

But here's the good news: Bias is not always bad, and better yet, it is sometimes quite helpful. There is bad bias, and there is beneficial bias. The key is to know which is which, and it's easier than you think.

At this point, I suspect you will pause for a moment, put your hand on your chin, gently frown, and say "hmm." If you are even a tiny bit cynical you will be questioning whether my bold comments about bias make sense: "Is it true that everyone is biased? And can this really work to my advantage?"

Yes and yes. Setting aside the negative connotation, what is a bias? To its holder, it is little more than an opinion that feels more like the objective truth than a subjective viewpoint. It is often based on carefully considered information and extensive experience. It may also be the result of a lifetime of exposure to the views of well-meaning influencers including educators, governments, media, parents, peers, and many others. Any point of view, ours and theirs, is unavoidably a product of our cumulative experience so far, inevitably leading to the beliefs, opinions, and biases we hold. This is our life. It is who we are. How can it be otherwise?

We express and encounter biases every day, often trivial ones. When I choose the Dutch apple cobbler drizzled with warm caramel, accompanied by a scoop of whole bean vanilla ice cream, the server might gleefully exclaim, "Good choice! That's my favorite and everyone loves it. It's the best item on the dessert menu!" Huh. Is it really?

Before we go too far astray, let's return to our man in the hot seat: Newt. Like you, he just read my intro to bias and is now lamenting the loss of an easy way out. He did not expect and does not want the seemingly daunting task of sifting through the sea of biased resources. Whether he knows it or not, Newt was hoping to find some sort of omniscient prostate cancer guru, maybe me, who would assimilate and correlate all aspects of his unique situation and then authoritatively tell him the one and only best road to take.

Newt wishes he could have an easy, definitive answer. Wouldn't that be lovely! Put a quarter in the slot, and out pops the message, "Your wish is granted." I'm not saying there is a connection here, but Newt is fantasizing about a scene from the classic movie *Big*, starring Tom Hanks. Have you seen it? Remember the powerful Zoltar machine? That's exactly what Newt wants, and his quarter is at the ready.

Well, despite how wonderful it would be, he knows Zoltar (it's real, look it up) cannot grant wishes and there is no omniscient prostate cancer guru. There may not even be just a single answer, but possibly more than one reasonable path to follow. Despite all this, Newt may still be tempted to bestow omniscience upon someone he trusts or allow a self-appointed guru to claim this mantle. Either way, the desired infallibility will be an illusion. We can hope that someday there will be a powerful computer program that will flawlessly analyze literally all possible avenues and outcomes, providing the best option every time. But not today, and probably not for a quarter.

Okay, that will suffice for generalities. Newt's "Bias 101" class is over. It's time to be specific, time to dig deeper. Despite how eager he is to hit the road and move forward, he must first look back and recall where it all began. Newt should now close his eyes, keep reading, take slow, deep breaths, and remember that fateful day when ... ah, yes ...

*♪ ♪Twinkling transition music plays softly
as the scene morphs into a now familiar setting ...*

Your friendly urologist

In his mind's eye, Newt's surroundings gradually come into focus. He remembers it clearly, a day that will live in infamy, his first encounter on the great prostate cancer adventure trail. In almost every case, the journey begins in the office of our friendly urologist. This lucky doctor is the one who usually breaks the news that yes indeed, the dreaded "C" word has been added to our personal lexicon.

"Ron, I have good news and bad news. The bad news is you have cancer," said mine, "but it's the good kind, it's early, and we can control it." Ugh? Yay? I'm so confused! How should I react to the warped pseudo-upbeat message delivered with such sincere optimism from Dr. Pee, as my urologist calls himself, saying "I'm just an old country pee doctor." That he is.

The key word from Dr. Pee was "early," and early detection is the goal. Thankfully, my primary physician was watching my PSA level, which can provide a clue, not a definitive diagnosis, that prostate cancer *might* be present. He also did an annual DRE (digital rectal exam), which is ironically an analog exam in which a finger is used to feel the prostate via the adjacent entryway alluded to in the very name of this quick, infamous procedure. When he became suspicious of my situation, he sent me to meet Dr. Pee.

I was lucky. With my routine PSA and DRE tests we caught it early. When the cancer is confined to the prostate and has not spread beyond, it is easiest to treat effectively. In later stages when it has already metastasized, treatment options are different. Once it has spread, therapy typically includes a systemic component such as hormone and/or chemotherapy for later-stage metastatic prostate cancer. Achieving a successful outcome is a more intense battle requiring heavier weapons, but still winnable.

Decisions are difficult with any prostate cancer diagnosis, and regardless of whether we caught it early, the road we travel is essentially the same. Along that road we will encounter bias, which brings us back to the topic at hand. Remember? We are in our urologist's office with Dr. Pee.

How did you respond to your pee doctor's news? The first follow-up question for most of us is obvious: "Okay, Doc, what should I do about it? How do I get rid of it?" That was my question, and Newt's. We instinctively wanted this doctor to be the final authority, our guru, our Zoltar. Just grant my wish, tell me what to do, and I'll do it so I can get on with my life. Hurry up. Tell me. Here's a quarter.

Now, this is where it gets interesting with some urologists. Nearly all of them are surgeons. They know how to remove a prostate and have probably done so many times successfully. They are justifiably proud of their surgical skills. You might hear them refer to surgery as "the gold standard" for treating prostate cancer. Should it surprise Newt when his urologist tells him he is a good candidate for surgery? "Let's schedule the procedure, cut it out, and move on." Yes! Yes! YES!

Newt's competent and experienced urologist—let's call him Dr. Kutter—clearly has a pro-surgery bias, which is understandable. He's an expert who spent years learning how to do it well and he has seen it work. He believes in surgery, is confident in his skill, and sincerely expects he will help Newt by removing his cancerous prostate. How could we expect him to think otherwise?

And yet some urologists do think otherwise, like Dr. Pee, one of the many exceptions to this pattern. Although he is a surgeon and said he would remove my prostate if I wanted him to, he did not believe a prostatectomy was the right choice for me. Amazing! He then scribbled a barely legible list of other options for me on a scrap of paper, briefly explaining the pros and cons of each. Proton therapy, often omitted from such lists, was included on his. He readily admitted not knowing much about proton therapy and was only vaguely aware of its advantages, yet he urged me to research it. I will forever be grateful to Dr. Pee for setting aside his knife and picking up a pen to produce this precious scrap of paper, and for his encouragement to investigate proton therapy.

While Dr. Pee was advising me to do some research, think it over, and let him know how I'd like to proceed, Dr. Kutter was already checking his surgical schedule, his pen in hand, ready to add Newt as soon as possible. For Dr. Pee, it was a *take a breath and think it over* approach. For Dr. Kutter, it was *let's get this show on the road!* With these responses, both demonstrated their respective biases, and make no mistake: both are biased. Knowing this, how should we respond?

The best strategy for using a bias to our advantage is to probe further into the reasons for it. When I asked Dr. Pee what he thought about radical prostatectomies in general and why he thought surgery was not the best choice for me, I learned quite a bit. Likewise, Newt should ask Dr. Kutter why he believes surgery is the gold standard, and which other modalities might also be effective and worth considering. He could also ask hypothetically which therapy would be a good second choice if he preferred not to have surgery.

In answering my questions, Dr. Pee demonstrated his rare-for-urologists bias against doing surgery if there are non-invasive alternatives with comparable or better outcomes. His bias is that surgery is a last resort, not an automatic first response. He also demonstrated a pro-patient bias by empowering me to have a significant role in deciding how to proceed and supporting me in whatever choice I made.

Dr. Kutter's answers for Newt were also kind, supportive, and informative about why he believes surgery is Newt's best option. Yet, to his credit and despite his strong pro-surgery bias, he made it clear that he will respect and stand by Newt even if alternatives are considered or chosen and will continue to serve as Newt's urologist through thick and thin, just like Dr. Pee does for me.

I hope your urologist will be as compassionate, patient-focused, and supportive as Dr. Kutter and Dr. Pee, but occasionally you might encounter a *my way or the highway* attitude. Although everyone, even doctors, are entitled to a strong opinion, the final decision is yours. If they cannot support your decision, expect a respectful professional referral to someone who can, rather than a *my-way / highway* ultimatum. In that case, the highway is sometimes the right choice.

And then there's the closely related matter of absolutes. The use of words like *always* and *never* is an easily identified reliable tipoff that a strong, barely hidden bias is lurking nearby. If you are told that men over sixty should *never* consider prostate surgery, that radiation *always* causes fatigue, that chemotherapy *always* offers the best chance of a cure, that hormone therapy *always* improves your outcome, that a holistic approach is *never* worth a try, that active surveillance is *always* a crazy idea, or that everyone *always* orders the caramel apple pie and they *never* regret it, then dismiss the advice as single-minded dogma and not particularly useful. Always.

There are pros and cons for all prostate cancer therapies, including surgery and proton therapy. If anyone tells you that surgery is archaic or that proton radiation is experimental, you might rightfully want a second opinion. Likewise, if you are told that surgery is always best or that proton has made all other therapies obsolete, you might again want to take the highway and seek a second opinion.

Newt finally made it out of Dr. Kutter's office, diagnosis in hand, and now it is time to move forward and tackle whatever comes next. Let the fun begin!

Okay. Not fun. Well, maybe a little. Sometimes.

Family, friends, and coworkers

After his lovely morning chat with Dr. Kutter, Newt heads back to his place of employment to finish his workday. He has an office job where the breakroom houses the proverbial water cooler, filled not with water, but with gossip juice. Based on recent interoffice underground communiques, everyone already suspects Newt may have prostate cancer. As Newt enters the office, Pat, the receptionist dutifully stops him to verify this. Newt confirms the diagnosis, and Pat quickly heads to the breakroom. Within mere milliseconds everyone knows.

Without exception, they are sorry Newt has prostate cancer and everyone would like to help. Many know that the only help they can provide is emotional support, which is extremely valuable and much appreciated. Of course, many of his coworkers also have an opinion about what Newt should do. Some will hide it and others will offer to share it. A few will attempt to impose it as the only course of action that makes sense.

The latter group is the smallest, but most vocal of the bunch. Fortunately, Newt has become good at politely letting them know he appreciates their viewpoint, values their concern, and will certainly consider their opinion. But regardless of how adamant they are, Newt must not feel obliged to follow their unqualified medical advice. He knows they mean well, but also knows they are not experts and their point of view is not expert guidance. Only experts are expert.

While there might be some valid and useful information in this avalanche of advice, only those educated in the field of medicine and prostate cancer can provide expert medical information. Treating cancer is a tricky proposition. Laymen certainly don't know how to do it. Even professionals disagree with each other, but regardless of differing medical viewpoints, an opinion from a doctor counts more than one from your friend's friend who is a barista at the corner coffee shop whose brother had prostate cancer three years ago.

At the end of the workday Newt goes home to find his wife, her sister, his brother, and their two best friends from next door sipping California Cabernet in the living room. They offer a glass to Newt as they turn toward him in unison, all sporting slightly forced smiles. "I'll bet you could use a drink," they say in various ways. They are right about that, but wrong about the Cab. He grabs a beer from the fridge.

Then, not unlike his experience at work, they all do their best to console and counsel Newt. This time he is well-prepared with a ready repertoire of responses rehearsed and tested with his coworkers. Newt easily sees the biases, and he accepts the sincere, well-intentioned comments for what they're worth, feeling fortunate to have the loving support of his family and friends.

His brother has taken all of this especially seriously because he loves his only sibling and because he knows there is a genetic component that increases his own chance of making prostate cancer a family tradition. He has already done some research and even bought a book recommended by a friend of his who had proton therapy last year. He hands the book to Newt.

Hey, look! It is the same book *you* are reading now. What a coincidence!

The author of this book (me)

As Newt borrows my book from his brother, and before you suffer bias burnout and skip the rest of this chapter (please don't), I should take the opportunity, more of an obligation, to come clean about my own bias. So far, I have discussed those commonly held by urologists, friends, family, and coworkers. Well, I am no exception to the "everyone is biased" axiom, so to avoid becoming a hypocrite, it seems proper to at least attempt full disclosure. Doing so will not eliminate my bias, but at least you will clearly know what it is, or at least what I think it is.

Here's my story, CliffsNotes style:

I was diagnosed with prostate cancer in late 2010 and to treat it I opted for **proton** beam radiation, not to be confused with the very different conventional x-ray (**pho**ton) radiation. I chose to receive this therapy in Jacksonville at the University of Florida Health Proton Therapy Institute, a leading facility among a handful (now dozens) of centers offering proton radiation for prostate and other cancers. Everyone at UF Proton was terrific, and even ten years later I am extremely pleased with the outcome. If your circumstances are similar to mine, I think you should do the same thing because it worked great for me. How could I think otherwise?

I am **pro-proton** and happy to say so.

This does not mean I am *anti-other-therapies* or *anti-other-facilities*. To treat prostate cancer today there is a Golden-Corral-sized buffet of ways to treat the nasty disease, and many great cancer treatment centers. In your research, you should independently evaluate and consider as many as you reasonably can. And as you read my book, please keep in mind that *my* biases are based on *my* research and *my* personal experience. I can't help it.

Here it is again: I am pro-proton. More precisely, here is what I mean by this short phrase that sounds like I'm stuttering: I strongly believe that you should at least be aware of proton beam therapy, study and consider it along with your other options, and ultimately understand exactly why you chose it or not. Unfortunately, it is sometimes not even mentioned to prostate cancer newbies and is therefore overlooked and not even considered. Your goal should be to compile a list of *all* options available, without ruling out any with a premature summary judgement. Give them all a fair chance and be clear about how and why you arrive at your final decision.

I will stick to The Game Plan and resist the temptation to digress into a full discussion of the unique characteristics and virtues of proton as compared with x-ray/photon radiation, not the topic of this book. Instead, I will boil it down to one mega-sentence:

> Unlike the **x-ray beam** of conventional radiation which radiates everything in its path including a lot of healthy tissue before and beyond its target, a **proton beam** deposits most of its payload at the target, with less radiation on the way to it and nothing measurable beyond it, thus minimizing exposure of healthy tissue to radiation and reducing the chance of side effects or secondary cancers later.

That's it in a nutshell. If you want the full unabridged version, please read my first book and completely uncensored story, *PROTONS versus Prostate Cancer: EXPOSED*. It is a detailed account of the patient's experience (mine) undergoing proton beam therapy. It's non-technical but thorough. Once you've read it, you will understand how proton therapy works, exactly what it's like to experience it, and why it should be considered.

Considered. It might not be right for you for medical reasons or personal ones, but by all means, ask your doctor if proton therapy is right for you. I know some prostate cancer patients who did not qualify for this therapy, and others who made valid alternative choices for a variety of individual reasons. Although I do not know any proton patients who wish they had done something else, I do understand that proton is not for everyone. But it absolutely should be considered.

To be perfectly precise, I am pro-*considering*-proton, or *pro-proton* for short.

That's my bias and I'm sticking to it.

And by the way, even *you* have one. Yours is the one that matters most, so don't ignore it.

Healthcare facilities

By now, I'm pretty sure you understand how biases pervade the entire process Newt faces. As he moves ahead following his D-Day (diagnosis day), he will bump into the biases we already discussed, plus others that might surprise him.

Diagnosis in hand, what's next for Newt? Conversations with ambassadors, which we have already analyzed in "The Newbie Trap" section, and a lot of research, which we'll discuss later. Soon enough, Newt will have a pretty good idea about which therapies and facilities he wants to consider, and he will begin contacting them.

At this early point in time, Newt was not yet sure whether proton therapy or some other type of treatment was the way to go. So, he contacted several reputable cancer centers with varying specialties, received their information, and even scheduled in-person consultations with three of his top candidates for treatment. Surely, he thought, this approach would illuminate the best path, the right one for Newt's unique situation, for curing his cancer with no side effects.

The result was now predictable to me, but not to Newt. All three centers—one specializing in brachytherapy, another in HIFU (high intensity focused ultrasound), and the third in proton therapy—wanted Newt. If we include Dr. Kutter, his urologist who had already made his case for surgery, there would be four totally different options. And wouldn't you know it, each declared Newt to be an ideal candidate for their form of treatment at their facility. How can this be?

Not surprisingly, the highly skilled medical professionals at these facilities are genuinely confident they can help Newt. They sincerely believe that their specialty is his best option and are not trying to mislead him. They have faith in themselves, their skill, their therapy, and their business. This conviction is the foundation of their bias, and although they may indeed be able to help Newt, they are not unbiased.

If we know this, we can use it to our advantage. Let the surgeon make the best possible argument for surgery; let the radiation oncologist present the case that radiation is best, and so on. Their bias is part of what we pay them for, and as long as we recognize it as such, we'll be able to interpret it accordingly and benefit from it. By giving each facility the chance to put its best foot forward, Newt can obtain great insight into the benefits of each treatment option.

Remember when I said not all bias is bad?

But wait, there's more! There is yet another type of bias Newt can use to his advantage. This one is a result of the indisputable fact that healthcare is a business. People in any business, including healthcare, must build and maintain a healthy, successful enterprise. Surgeons, radiologists, clinics, and hospitals who are no longer in business are of no value to Newt in his battle with cancer. Even the purest among them understand that they must offer more than just expertise. To remain profitable and keep their doors open, they must also find enough people who want their expertise. So of course, they want *you* and they want you to want them. Isn't that nice!

This means there is competition for your business as a cancer patient (or customer, as crude as it may sound), although it might be more fashionable and politically correct to deny this, or at least leave it unstated. Surgeons compete with each other, radiologists compete with each other, surgeons compete with radiologists, and so on. A growing number of proton therapy centers want and need your business to stay afloat, too, and although they cooperate with each other, they must also compete.

I'm not saying they are happy you have cancer. Certainly not. I am merely pointing out that they want you to choose them to treat it. And unless they are sure they absolutely cannot help you, they will want you to give them a chance. They want your business.

They even advertise, which still strikes me as a little weird even though it shouldn't. Have you noticed those billboards along the interstates promoting prostate cancer treatment? You know, the ones that are often right next to the smiling personal injury lawyer with a cool slogan and symmetrical phone number? Such billboards should remind you that curing cancer is a competitive business. The main reason cancer centers spend big money to deliver their message is to win your business instead of watching you go elsewhere.

Remember, ads are not public service announcements, and although they are required to be truthful, they are not objective. Ads are designed to help gain your trust, your confidence, and your business. And yes, they also want and need your money (or that of your insurance company).

After all this time and effort Newt is more confused than ever, but he should be happy there is competition for his business. Competitors will have to do what any successful business must do: provide a first-rate service at a competitive price and present a convincing argument that you should choose them. Let's hope the competition continues to be vigorous and rigorous.

And let's hope Newt can sort it all out and make a good decision, never needing to call that lawyer.

Beyond the bias.

Poor Newt. He has gradually embraced the notion that everyone is biased. He now understands that prostate cancer treatment is a competitive business. But how can he sort through this mess? He knows he needs help and he very much wants to trust *someone*, but how can he know who to trust?

Let's help Newt figure this out by using a system of points. Trust points. TPs.

If an individual or facility is highly regarded, has years of experience, offers unfiltered references (e.g., a voluntary ambassador list), and seems to genuinely care, that's perfect. Learn as much as you can from them. If their information proves to be consistently valid and useful, they will eventually earn your confidence. This kind of trust is quite valuable and worth 10 TPs. Write it down.

But be wary of sources who have an answer for everything. It may seem ironic, but I always find it to be refreshing and confidence-engendering to hear someone state unashamedly that they do not know something. "I don't know" is a phrase we do not hear very often, and when we do, we may react with disappointment. But it is the best answer we can hope for when it is the truth.

Again, I will reference my urologist Dr. Pee, the surgeon who first told me about proton therapy. Remember him? When I asked him to tell me more about how proton differs from conventional IMRT he told me what little he knew, and readily admitted he did not know much about it. Nevertheless, he felt it was worth my time to investigate further and encouraged me to do so. Imagine that! A surgeon, urging me to explore proton beam therapy! At that moment his trust quotient rose significantly, and I began listening to him even more carefully. Today he remains one of my most trusted physicians.

You can award 3 TPs for each time you hear a sincere "I don't know." Dr. Pee eventually earned 30 points in this category and he adds to it every time I see him. But watch out for three or more consecutive eyes-closed headshaking "I don't knows." This is just worthless fretting, and not point-worthy.

On the flipside of the previous point category, you should deduct 5 TPs for any substantial conversation in which you do not even once hear "I don't know" or something similar. This is called a *know-it-all penalty*. It can only be invoked if you ask a lot of questions, as you should.

Next, even after reading "The Newbie Trap" section, Newt asks, "What about points for prostate cancer patients who have already had therapy? After all, we're on the same team, so to speak, so can we automatically trust them?"

Regardless of the type of therapy, if you ask a man how it went, he'll likely say it was somewhere between pretty well and great. Unlike product reviews in which hordes of buyers love to publicly complain about toasters and such, prostate cancer survivors tend to emphasize the positive. After all, we're still here! Along with a past patient's bias for the positive, his comments might not always be directly related to his treatment at all, but rather to his well-being when you ask, even if it has no relationship whatsoever to the therapy.

So, how should we award trust points to ambassadors? Let's give each the benefit of a doubt and start with 5 TPs. However, if they never make a negative comment or never make a positive one, deduct 4 of those points because no therapy can be 100% perfect or 100% horrible. If they have written a book on the subject give them 2 bonus points for making the effort. Ambassadors who are scientists would be expected to use clear, objective thinking, and deserve 3 bonus points if they do. Those in the medical field—and we know that even urologists and oncologists can get prostate cancer—earn 4 bonus TPs for a willingness to share their personal experience along with their unique insider's point of view, a rare and valuable combination.

Still, Newt will not find any single source he can count on to tell him everything about everything. It remains up to him to determine in which specific areas each credible source can be trusted, and to pay close attention to what they say about that. Only Newt can separate the trustworthy information from the rest, and only he can decide which sources offer at least some reliable information.

People do want to help and are usually sincere, and if they had no bias they wouldn't be human. It is up to us to puzzle together a reasonably complete picture, even with all the bias, and then choose a path. When all is said and done, we must trust our own assessment and instincts. We have to trust ourselves, and if Newt can do that, he gets a whopping 50 trust points and wins the game! By the way, Newt is making a list:

(1) Everyone is biased.
(2) Only experts are expert.
(3) Trust must be earned.

One, two, three. See how simple it is?

Not.

RISK, TIMING, AND DECISIONS

Newt has his diagnosis. He has survived an avalanche of advice from friends, family, coworkers, and nearly everybody on planet Earth. On his desk there are stacks of packets of information from cancer centers. In his browser he has bookmarked lots of links to informative websites. On his bookshelf, previously dominated by Stephen King, Lee Child, and Dr. Seuss, there is now a special section for books like this one.

In his head there is chaos and confusion. Poor Newt! What is he to do? Well, it's another one-two-three step deal. Here it is:

Assess the risks,
decide what to do and when to do it,
and then do it.

Assess. Decide. Do
1 -2 - 3

Easy to say, hard to accomplish.

What makes it so hard?

It's the risks. If there were none, it would be easy. The justification for taking a risk is the promise of reward, and whether it's worth it or not is totally subjective.

There are people who thrive on the thrill of risky maneuvers in finance, business, sports, and so on. But when it comes to health, especially when a life-threatening issue is perceived, most of us try to avoid risks, especially big ones but also small ones.

I take very few big risks, real or imagined. A big one that paid off nicely was marrying Lucy. She wasn't the risk, but I was petrified of marriage, which felt like diving into the deep end without a clue about swimming. Thankfully, after taking the plunge, she taught me to swim.

I often take smaller risks than marriage. For example, pizza. Lucy and I are fussy. We like our pizza well-done to the point where mere mortals would consider it ruined. We have about a 50-50 chance of getting it that way. We can live with the risk of suffering a substandard pizza because when they get it right, it's great.

Prostate cancer is more serious than pizza, but also risky. In choosing a plan of action, we all share the hope of curing the cancer with no side effects. We also share the fear that doing the wrong thing at the wrong time can end badly, with little chance for a do-over another day. The more likely outcome is somewhere in the middle, but our focus at the outset is on the extremes.

Newt does not want to die of prostate cancer, nor does he want to ruin his current symptom-free good life in exchange for defeating the cancer. I understand this challenge because I faced it in 2010. It is a daunting dilemma requiring an understanding of not only these current risks, but of our personal tolerance for risk in general. The latter can be hard to define. How much risk is acceptable? What kind are we most comfortable with?

No doubt about it, this is a complex situation, and making sense of it can feel overwhelming.

Let's help Newt figure it out.

Risk is unavoidable.

Life is full of risky situations. Action involves risk. Inaction involves risk, as well. I will not digress into the all-time favorite "you risk your life every time you drive your car" speech. The relevant fact here is that with a cancer diagnosis we are saddled with new risks, and there is nothing we can do about it. For you, me, and Newt, they have now become a fact of life.

When you have prostate cancer, on any given day you have the same choice: you can treat it or not. Either way, there are risks. There is no way out, so Newt might as well get busy wrapping his brain around his new reality. And the sooner the better because although it can feel scary, once confronted, you and Newt will see the light at the end of the tunnel where everything usually turns out fine.

Quick review question: Exactly why is treating prostate cancer so risky?

Brief answer: Because the bladder sits atop it; the rectum brings up the rear; the urethra (the tube from the bladder) goes directly through it; the cavernous nerves (controlling erection) surround it. Treating a cancerous prostate without affecting the bladder, rectum, urethra, or nerves is all but unimaginable. Yet this is precisely the goal of every therapy: kill the cancer in the prostate without bothering the neighboring healthy tissue. No small undertaking.

Most treatment options are getting better at approaching this seemingly impossible goal, but none are perfect. In this anatomical minefield, no treatment can make any guarantees, the risk of any given side effect is never zero, and the specific risks vary from one therapy to another. To further complicate matters, some therapies have lower cancer recurrence rates than others. Plus, all treatments do not have the same success rate for controlling the cancer in the first place, which is arguably the main job. It's complicated.

To make matters even trickier, there can be concern about whether cancer cells have traveled out of the prostate, beyond the so-called capsule around it. Depending on the likelihood of this in your circumstances, you might want to target areas beyond the prostate to kill any renegade cells just outside the capsule. But doing this might increase the risk of collateral damage. Did I mention that it's complicated?

"Okay, okay, okay," says Newt. "I get it. I cannot avoid risk, and it's complicated. One way or the other, I'm stuck with it and might as well face it head-on."

And he's right. Facing this head-on is the best approach. It is a delicate balancing act, and no one can tell him how to weigh the risk of treatment-related side effects against the risk of allowing his cancer to progress at an indeterminable pace. Truth be told—and truth-telling is highly recommended—maybe Newt doesn't care as much about certain side effects as some people think he should. Maybe he doesn't care about the cancer as much as some others think they would if they were in his shoes. That's fine, but they are not in his shoes. Newt is the one who must assess the risks and live with the results.

With a prostate cancer diagnosis, your challenge is to determine which approach strikes the right balance in a way that fits your unique life, and there is no right or wrong about this highly personal choice. For example, if you are not sexually active then the risks associated with sexual function may not influence your decisions. If you have other serious health issues or are lucky enough to already be very old, you might find the risks of deferring treatment more acceptable than those of therapy-related collateral damage that could negatively impact the quality of your remaining years.

There is no 100% risk-free winning strategy, so do not expect to find one. All you can do is weigh the known risks and choose a reasonable path forward. This is not the first time you have confronted life's risks, and it won't be the last. You can handle it, and things will probably turn out just fine.

Timing is tricky.

I remember quite well the instant sense of urgency my diagnosis injected into my life. I could feel the clock ticking as never before, and time is certainly not our friend with respect to cancer.

The cancer cells are not likely to suddenly disappear or become magically benign, and if left unchecked, there will probably not be fewer cancer cells tomorrow than today. I felt like I was in a race against time.

But as Dr. Pee reminded me, *prostate* cancer often, but not always, progresses slowly, especially as compared with other forms of cancer, and it is usually not imminently life-threatening. Knowing this can be either good or bad. It allowed me time to adequately understand my situation and options, and that's good. But it could have lulled me into becoming a perpetual research machine, endlessly seeking but never quite having enough information to make decisions, which is bad. Fortunately, I avoided falling down the rabbit hole of research, one of my favorite places where I am usually quite content.

Are you old enough to remember Jack Benny? As far as I know, the late comedian did not have prostate cancer, but he understood timing. With a gun pointed at Jack, the robber demands, "Your money or your life!" After a long minute with no response, he impatiently repeats more loudly, "Look, bud. Your money or your life?" Benny puts his hand on his cheek, slowly turns his head away from the robber, and shouts with annoyance, "I'm thinking it over!"

Most of us have the luxury of leisurely thinking it over, but not all of us. If your prostate cancer is more aggressive, has spread, or is late-stage, you may want to delay little in choosing an approach that will buy you as much quality time as possible. Ironically, you will also become highly motivated to do what many people without cancer fail to do: Get busy living your life. Just like everyone else, you still have the rest of your life ahead of you, and just like everyone else, you don't know how much time you'll have. But unlike the rest, you have had a wake-up call to dust off that bucket list and start checking things off. Not a bad idea for any of us.

Thankfully, with early diagnosis of prostate cancer becoming increasingly common, this urgent scenario is not typical. In most cases we might reasonably expect to live many more years, even decades, until something else inevitably gets us. When caught early, prostate cancer can likely be cured or controlled effectively by more than one therapy, but the cure rates and side effects can vary. It therefore makes sense to take a reasonable amount of time to evaluate not only the potential quantity of life, but also the quality of life afforded by each course of action.

There is a potential tradeoff between quantity and quality. While cancer threatens to shorten the amount of life remaining, every treatment threatens to reduce your quality of life during that time. Sometimes we delay treatment hoping to postpone facing this possible tradeoff, forgetting that these are merely threats, not promises. There is also the possibility of no compromise at all: no more cancer with no side effects. This is a scenario we can hope for *if* we do the right thing at the right time.

"But," asks Newt, "why do anything at all? I have no symptoms and I feel fine!"

Great question. Prostate cancer often has no symptoms until its later stages. With early diagnosis, the perceived risk of collateral damage from treatment is magnified by the fact that you may feel just fine today. Newt feels fine, so he naturally wonders why he should rock the boat. Seems like whatever he might do, he can only make it worse.

Of course, that's not true because he can't see the cancer cells or what they're doing. Things can definitely get worse. However, prostate cancer does allow the sometimes very reasonable option to wait and see how it develops: active surveillance. But the timing is tricky. The longer you wait, the more difficult treatment might become, and the more risk you might have to face later with less attractive future options. Might. Might. And might not.

Newt has fully digested all of this discussion of timing, and as usual, he has the perfect question. He wants to know how to come out on top. How should he play his cards? With the hand he's been dealt, what's the right play? The good news for Newt is that the deck is stacked in his favor. No matter what he does, he is likely to win, or at least draw.

Here's the deal for Newt, and for you: If you delay treatment and die from something else before experiencing debilitating symptoms of prostate cancer, **you win** the bet. Or if you treat and cure the cancer with tolerable or no side effects, **you have hit the jackpot**. If you let the cancer run its course and later develop a high-risk advanced cancer with serious symptoms, it could still be **a win for you**, depending on how long it is before that happens and what medical advances have been made in the interim. And finally, if you treat and control the cancer now but are unhappy with your side effects (whatever they might be), you will have lost some quality but gained quantity, so **it's a draw**. The only way cancer wins is if your course of action (or inaction) is totally ineffective at both controlling it and avoiding symptoms or side effects, a relatively uncommon result in today's world. All in all, the odds are heavily in your favor.

Cancer or not, timing is tricky. How much remaining quality time will you have? No one knows and having prostate cancer does not endow you with or entitle you to that knowledge. Just do your less-than-perfect best to understand your options, and then weigh the risks relative to your personal quantity-versus-quality priorities and your tolerance for risk, as only you can.

A decision is unavoidable.

It is easy to slip into perpetual procrastination when the fear of making a wrong decision is great. I am a lifelong procrastinator and I like to get things right, a debilitating combination. When my toaster recently died, I endured several no-toast months while I researched every toaster on the market before I was sufficiently confident about which would fulfill my toasting expectations. As you can imagine, back in 2010 my fear of choosing the wrong cancer therapy was extreme when I was faced with new, important, life-changing decisions that make toaster shopping seem easy, if not trivial.

You can research, consider, contemplate, discuss, and scratch your head endlessly about how to proceed. But from the moment you were diagnosed, you were forced into the first and most fundamental decision: Will you be proactive, reactive, or passive in addressing your cancer diagnosis? There is no avoiding this decision because like it or not, the default is being passive, letting the chips fall where they may.

Now it becomes a bit more subtle. At this point, an inevitable series of decisions are in motion, culminating in the final big decision about whether to postpone therapy or to schedule a particular treatment now. You will begin with the decision to research your options. You will decide how to conduct your research: websites, books, professional publications, professionals, friends, patients, etc. You'll make decisions about how much each source of information can be trusted and which information matters most. And you should, but might not decide how much time you will devote to research before making your final decision.

Well, fellow toaster shoppers, here's the rub: if you don't draw a somewhat arbitrary line in the sand for making that final decision, you risk perpetual procrastination. Seth Godin, one of my favorite modern philosophers, makes this astute observation about drawing that line:

> *The deluge that is the internet is an opportunity and a problem. With a few clicks, we're able to get more data. And there's no end in sight, since new data is posted faster than we can consume it. ... It's easy to be in favor of more data. After all, until we reach a certain point, more data is the best way to make a better decision. But then, fairly suddenly, more isn't better. It's simply a way to become confused or to stall.*
>
> [from *Seth's Blog*, https://seths.blog/2021/08/controlling-information/]

Without consciously setting a reasonably finite timeline you will have inadvertently accepted the default decision to research indefinitely, to stall, even if you have not acknowledged or even realized this. Endlessly seeking just one more bit of data is a dangerous slippery slope, probably motivated by the fear of missing something relevant. But missing something is guaranteed because the moment you believe you have a consensus about a particular toaster, someone will post a new review with additional insight, or worse yet, new models will be introduced.

Continuing research is a decision to postpone treatment, even when disguised as a series of decisions to do *just a little more* research and gather a bit more data. Dropping the pretense that you are still deciding reveals the truth that you have in effect chosen the option of *watchful waiting*. There might be nothing wrong with this, but it should be a conscious choice, not accidental.

You can also just do nothing, not even research, but even that is a decision: it is the decision to be inactive and let nature take its course. The alternative is to take this bull by the horns and chart your own course, making timely decisions at each juncture. Either way, you will have decided. It is unavoidable.

The natural fear of making the wrong decision might paralyze you, and the fear of overlooking something could put you in perpetual research mode. But you can ignore the fear, and when you feel *reasonably* confident that you have *sufficient* information, make a decision and move forward. This is not the first challenge you've faced, nor will it be the last, and you can handle it.

Newt still looks confused, so let me succinctly sum it up: (1) Action and inaction are both decisions. (2) Deciding not to decide is a decision. (3) Delaying a decision is a decision. (4) It is impossible to avoid making a decision.

Go ahead. Buy a toaster.

There are good treatment options today

When it comes to *prostate* cancer, there is a lot of good news.

With today's science and technology, most prostate cancer can be cured or significantly controlled. Early diagnosis is always best, but there are effective therapies even with a late diagnosis. There are options, combinations of options, and variations on each option. The smorgasbord of therapy for prostate cancer is dazzling, which also makes it confusing and difficult to choose, but the sometimes-forgotten point is that there are many good options now.

Surgery has become increasingly high-tech and promises better outcomes today than a decade ago. Hormone therapy and chemotherapy have improved and are often combined with other modes of treatment in creative ways. Even conventional photon/x-ray radiation now includes many innovative delivery strategies aimed at reducing radiation damage to other organs.

Proton radiation, a newer, very different, well-established technology, can even further minimize radiation exposure to healthy tissue by virtue of its unique Bragg Peak effect: lower radiation levels upon entry, maximum at the target, and no radiation on exit. And current advances in proton therapy promise even better cure rates with fewer side effects.

Remember, I'm a proton ambassador. You saw my card.

I had some incredibly good treatment options in 2010, as you do now. Today, regardless of when your today may be, you also have the good fortune of being able to choose between some very effective treatments, each with different characteristics, and most with a good chance of success.

You can confidently go forth and conquer. Choose your weapon, fight the monster, and win the battle.

There will be new therapies tomorrow.

Newt has been paying close attention, but I fear I have given him the wrong idea. I can tell what he is thinking because I know him well. Newt is thinking, *my cancer was caught early, I have no symptoms, Ron said therapies are improving rapidly. Maybe I should move my line in the sand, hang in there a while longer, and wait for some newer, better approach. Sit tight and hope for the silver bullet.*

There is no need for Newt to wonder if there will be better options tomorrow for someone in his shoes. There will. But it is a mistake to use that certainty as a reason to wait. To be sure, waiting is a legitimate choice and can sometimes be the right one, but not because of future options that don't yet exist.

Who knows, maybe one day there will be a 100% cure with no risk, or maybe even a vaccine. This possible future can be exciting to imagine but has little relevance to Newt today. What is similarly interesting and 100% relevant to Newt, is that he has much better options for dealing with his cancer today than he would have had ten or twenty years ago. Newt can be happy that his cancer occurred now, not then.

Think of it like this: Suppose you need a cell phone. Would you buy today's iPhone 13 when you can be pretty sure there will soon be an even better iPhone 14? But then, what will you do once the 14 has been released and the rumors about the 15 have begun, aaaaand you'll never buy a phone at all. Year after year, technology, including cancer therapy, will predictably and relentlessly improve, and the fear of missing out, sometimes referred to as FOMO, can leave you unable to make your move.

If some new data or procedure is announced soon after you complete your treatment of choice, you might wish you had waited a little longer and been able to take advantage of that development, but so what? There are many things in life for which hindsight is 20-20, and you cannot predict the future. Nor should you gamble recklessly with your future, unless you are the reckless gambling type, comfortable with that approach. More on that topic later.

I want to be perfectly clear that waiting is not the problem. Waiting because of anticipating buyer's remorse is the problem. If you have evaluated your situation and decided that the risk of active surveillance is reasonable, then fine: watch and wait. But if you are waiting because you are afraid that whatever you do today will be outdone by a better option tomorrow, you will find yourself waiting forever. You cannot allow yourself to become paralyzed by FOMO of inevitable advances.

You don't have cancer in the future; you have it today.

Today is yesterday's future, and with it came better cancer therapy options for you. Tomorrow is someone else's future and will undoubtedly afford even better options for them.

Now a decade later for me, I am in my own future and would still likely choose proton therapy. I'm glad I didn't wait ten years to do it, despite knowing now that it is even more effective today than it was then. If I had waited, I might have needed only half as many proton zaps. I might have never even heard of the infamous rectal balloon. The targeting of my cancer might have been a bit better with pencil beam technology, which was not an option in 2010. Even the lighting and music in the gantry will have improved. Golly gee, I sure wish my prostate cancer diagnosis had been in today's wonderful world!

But it was not. Prostate cancer knocked on my door in 2010.

PERFECTION AND PERSPECTIVE

Newt is a diligent fellow who does his best to do things right and to do the right things. Anyone who knows him would expect Newt to do his level best to approach prostate cancer correctly, which is exactly what he endeavors to do. Simply stated, he wants to do the best thing, the best way, at precisely the right time. Avoiding mistakes is important to Newt not only for these reasons, but also because he does not want to later hear what he should have done—a better approach, if only he had known.

When it comes to his prostate cancer, Newt will expend great energy and leave no stone unturned in pursuit of perfection. Where there's a will there's a way, and Newt is as determined as a politician in November.

If you are anything like Newt, then settle down in your easy chair with a hot cup of herbal tea. It's time to get real about a few things.

Like it or not ...

<u>No outcome will be perfect.</u>

Today as I write, there is no treatment guaranteed to cure prostate cancer. There is no therapy that does not carry at least some risk of undesirable side effects. There is no approach without a financial cost, and none without an investment of time and possibly some inconvenience.

Alas, there is no perfect answer and there will be no perfect outcome. The magic pill has not yet been found. No perfect pill, no silver bullet.

Although you may be saying, "Yeah, yeah, yeah, I already know this," do you accept it? Are you behaving as if you do?

I mention this again not to be discouraging, but to encourage you to avoid wasting valuable time on a wild goose chase. A universally correct perfect answer simply does not exist. Your time will be better spent determining a reasonable course of action. In today's world, there are likely several that can give you excellent outcomes. But not perfect, and that's okay.

No comprehensive study exists.

Time-waster #1 is seeking perfection. Time-waster #2 is searching for the study with all the answers.

Sure, there are tons of studies about cancer therapy, and some good ones with limited scope. But the one Newt most wants does not exist. There is no all-encompassing comprehensive study. This may not surprise you, but newbies do seem to have difficulty embracing this fact. After all, it is exactly what we all want: an analysis showing which treatment comes out on top, plain and simple. Is that asking too much? It's what I wanted when I was a newbie. It's what Newt wants. And I'll bet you do, too.

I am guessing that nearly every man who has had prostate cancer made a valiant effort to find a recent and reputable comparison of the risk/cure percentages of *all* available treatment options. If found, we could easily review the numbers and pick the winner. Well, let me save you some time: it doesn't exist and never will. How could it? It's a moving target. If you created an ambitious and all-inclusive list of options to compare, a new therapy would come along before your comparison was complete. You would be better off spending your time, effort, and energy elsewhere where you can be successful.

Elsewhere, like where? Maybe go to the ice cream parlor where you can create your own perfect concoction of scoops and toppings (hmm, I'll be right back). Guaranteed success!

Although you will not find the massive comparative study that can never exist, you can find many good, relevant studies providing helpful conclusions about specific topics. Of course, to varying degrees, they will all be out of date, but that's okay. Oddly, this latter point is good news. They are out of date because medical technology, like all technology, evolves and improves very fast. So fast that today's studies, typically requiring years to complete, are almost instantly yesterday's news. But those studies do have immense value. Oncology leaders learn from them and apply the knowledge to further improve the latest methodology. This means increasingly better results for us. We win!

Newt is smiling. He likes to win. He is energized and eager to return to his research, and is quickly ready with his next question: "Ron, how will I know which studies are useful? There are so many!"

It's a challenge, and there are seemingly countless studies to consider. Just as today's many remedies and facilities for treating prostate cancer will soon be joined by new ones, the opportunities for comparative studies will expand, and there will be an abundance of studies of all kinds. By matching any two or more items from a long list of available criteria, a study can be created. As you can imagine, the number of combinations of legitimate comparisons is already enormous and will continue to grow.

That's why Newt's question is a good one, not to be dismissed, so let's narrow it down. What should you watch for when considering the value of any given study? Let's consider an example.

Suppose you wanted to find a definitive analysis revealing whether surgery or proton therapy is more effective at curing prostate cancer. On the surface, this is a simple question comparing only two options. But without more detail within each of those two criteria, you could not make a valid personal decision based on such a vastly oversimplified generalized result.

You would be left wondering: Was the conclusion valid for all men, or only for those in a certain age bracket? Or only for men with a particular medical history (e.g., smoker, diabetic, high cholesterol, hypertension, prior cancers)? Or taking certain medications? With a specific PSA level, Gleason score, or staging at diagnosis? And so on. Plus, it would be unclear whether the study was valid for all variations of surgery (e.g., open surgery, laparoscopic, robotic) and all variations of proton therapy (e.g., scatter beam, pencil beam, total dosage, number of zaps). What about variations from one treatment center to another, or one country versus others, or treatment on Earth versus the Moon or Mars? [I include the latter in case you are reading this in the distant future.]

A comprehensive study would have to include all of the above, and more. What about recurrence in five, ten, twenty, or more years? What about patient-reported satisfaction, an important indication of post-treatment quality of life? This subjective measurement would need to be obtained following treatment at one, five, ten, or twenty years out. It should also include a breakdown of quality of life components: urinary function, sexual function, fatigue, and so on. So many questions! Endless combinations! And every one of them would be interesting and potentially useful in some way.

Let me be perfectly clear: I am not encouraging you to hunt for all this information, nor to seek studies cross-tabulating the virtually unlimited combinations of data. Just the opposite. Find a few personally pertinent, clearly defined, well-executed studies, each with limited scope.

There will be no shortage of useful analyses to digest, but there will be no single study with THE answer. So, find *some* relevant data, interpret it with the proper personal perspective, and use what you can. Try not to slide down the rabbit hole looking for the mother-of-all-studies. It doesn't exist.

Now let's go get some ice cream. I'll see you there.

All studies are not equally useful.

Newt is undeterred. He is committed to finding those potentially useful analyses I just mentioned. This begs a new and very reasonable question, which Newt is quick to ask: "How will I know if a study is a good one?" Good question. There is a lot to consider when evaluating the worthiness of a study.

I'm going to quote Seth Godin for the second time because he is super-smart:

> ... it's worth thinking hard about what it means for there to be a good study. Did they show their work? Have reputable peers referred to the study? What does the person publishing the study have to gain?
>
> [from *Seth's Blog*, https://seths.blog/2022/08/a-good-study/]

Seth's three questions are good food for thought. Let's unpack them in reverse order.

His last one ties in directly with bias, which we've already discussed at length. Organizing and conducting a study is no small matter. It requires time, money, a strong commitment, and a lot of hard work. No one in their right mind would undertake such a project without an expectation of a beneficial result, which is their reason for doing the study. This does not negate its potential value—it can still be a good study—but knowing the motive will help Newt identify any bias, allowing him to interpret the structure and conclusions with proper perspective. Ford would not survey pickup truck owners hoping to prove people prefer Chevy, and if that were their survey's conclusion you might never hear about it at all.

Next, Newt can legitimately wonder whether anybody else seems to care about the study, particularly the "reputable peers" Seth mentions. If there have been notable citations by respected sources, those will often be listed along with the study. If Ford's survey was comprehensive and objective with worthwhile conclusions, Consumer Reports might cite it, giving it greater credence.

If you don't regularly follow Seth Godin you might not know what he means by "show their work." Think back to your algebra class. If you could mentally solve for X and state the correct answer, you might only earn partial credit. For full credit, you would also need to provide all the steps leading to your solution: *your work*. Newt would be ill-advised to depend on a study unless it fully explained how it was conducted, how the underlying data was obtained, and how the conclusion was reached.

At the mention of data, Newt recalls that prostate cancer treatment is a diverse and competitive business. As much as we might wish otherwise, the competitors do not freely share all data, nor should they be expected to. This means Facility A may have access to some, but not all data from Facility B for inclusion in their analyses. Furthermore, if both facilities conduct similar, but independent studies, the underlying criteria might vary enough to make a direct apples-to-apples comparison difficult. Even if only the year differs in otherwise similar studies, valid comparisons may be nearly impossible. Would a Ford survey comparing their current year's pickups with Chevy's 1990 trucks be meaningful?

There are many worthwhile questions relating to a survey's underlying data. Was the sample large enough to be meaningful? Did the study accrue data in a prospective way? Or were conclusions drawn from existing historical data such as information obtained from public (i.e., government) insurance databases? Were patients periodically surveyed to provide meaningful subjective ratings of their post-treatment health? Were post-treatment follow-up medical diagnostics used? All of these are legitimate when clearly identified and used properly, but it is up to us to be aware of the nature of the data.

And then there is the techno-lingo, the terminology. Identical phrases might mean different things from different sources. For example, a study might offer a statistic concerning the frequency of minor, moderate, or severe "urinary complications" after treatment. But how is that determined? What exactly constitutes a complication? How is a minor one distinguished from a moderate or severe one? A study may use generally accepted definitions, but there is no requirement to do so. When definitions can vary, comparisons are challenging at best.

To summarize: It will be difficult if not impossible to compare one study to another if they are not using the same methodology, terminology, and measurement criteria. The year in which each study was conducted is also critically important for relevance and comparisons, so use your yellow highlighter (physical ones for paper reports, digital ones for computers) to clearly mark each date. Note the various data sources and the differing sample sizes. And be aware of not only the stated purpose, but also any possible hidden agenda and how it may affect the conclusions.

And now please dust off your crystal ball for a necessary look into your future.

Your perspective will change.

I cannot count the number of times I have said *if only I had known then what I know now!* But alas, life moves only forward. We are a blank slate at the start and have the greatest wisdom when we bid farewell. It can be a fun exercise to imagine this working in reverse, as in the movie *The Curious Case of Benjamin Button* (2008), but life is not a fantasy flick.

In high school I was socially paralyzed, unable to ask a girl on a date. Why? As I remember this period, it was fear of rejection, embarrassment, and feeling silly afterward. Somehow, I gradually became a bit bolder, not caring so much about rejection or humiliation. Thankfully, my new perspective arrived before Lucy did, or I could have cheated myself out of decades of loving her.

Similarly, what seems monumentally important to Newt today will very possibly seem much less so a year from now. Likewise, what will seem important in a few years might not even be on his radar today. This discrepancy is important because to make good decisions today he must anticipate how his perspective and priorities will have changed later. This is not easy for me, Newt, or you, and it is worth a closer look.

The first big issue is time, and specifically, the duration of your treatment. Some are relatively short, some take longer, and others are ongoing. The biggest conflict arises if the therapy you believe to be best for you takes notably longer than others. How can you possibly consider taking weeks off from work, going away from home, and leaving your normal responsibilities behind? How can life go on without you? Even if you believe that a prostate cancer treatment requiring weeks is your best medical option, you might conclude that you simply cannot afford to devote that amount time to treatment. Certainly not when there are quicker therapies available. And you might be right.

I have finally seen and accepted that the world *can* survive without me (and you) for days, weeks, or even months. At some point the world will have to find its way without you and me forever. Edison is gone, but the lights are still on. We are not as indispensable or irreplaceable as we might think or wish. We tend to have an inflated, even borderline-arrogant view of our importance, but that's not reality. If we have lived well, we naturally feel, and probably are, important to something or someone, but we are not indispensable.

I was facing this issue when I was still gainfully employed as the IT Training Coordinator for Richland County, South Carolina. When I started in that position in 2002 there was barely a hint of a coherent technology training program for county employees, and over the years I built a comprehensive and successful one I was quite proud of. And of course, I believed my personal involvement was critical, which I have now learned is utterly false. In 2011 the county survived my two months of proton therapy, and when I retired in 2015, Richland County Government forged ahead quite well without me. Sad, but true. Life goes on, even without not-so-indispensable me, for a little while or for good. Retirement is a humbling experience that brings a new perspective to life.

This is not to say our responsibilities and obligations don't matter. They do, and in meeting them we will find varying degrees of flexibility ranging from none to considerable. If you are fortunate to have some flexibility, temporary arrangements can often be made for managing things in your absence with the help of those who care. Taking the necessary time for your preferred treatment now will help ensure that you can resume your usual responsibilities later. Inconvenient or logistically challenging as it may be, investing more time today might be the best long-term strategy and is certainly worth exploring carefully rather than dismissing prematurely.

What about money? If you have insurance that will pay the whole bill for the treatment you prefer, there is no issue. If you don't, or if you would have some out-of-pocket cost for the therapy you have judged to be best for you, then you will have to determine how much you can afford. Would you take a second mortgage on your house? Sell your boat? Dip into your savings? Accept help from relatives?

If you find all these options impossible or undesirable, would you instead opt for what you consider to be your second choice, but more affordable treatment? Going with a perfectly viable Plan B may be fully justified if your financial resources are limited. If you decide to go with Plan B for this reason, do so confidently, with a commitment to never second-guess your decision later.

As you think about which financial resources you are willing to use, your level of commitment to obtaining your first-choice treatment will become clearer. I would love to have a top-of-the-line Tesla in my driveway, but instead I have a perfectly reliable Ford that gets me where I want to go. In a pawn shop, I recently saw a 1954

Gibson guitar I would love to have, and I could have tried to justify letting go of the big buckeroos to buy it. But I didn't, and I am perfectly happy with the instruments I am lucky enough to already have. Sometimes the second choice, Plan B, can be the right one.

And remember that like time, the money may well matter a lot less later than it does now. People often ask me what my housing expense was in Jacksonville in 2011, but I can't remember. What I do recall is that it seemed like a lot at the time. Now, it's just a forgotten number.

Whether you have ample or more limited resources and flexibility, it is entirely possible that your perspective will change later. To be sure, time and money are ongoing concerns for many people. But one or both might matter less in hindsight than you think, and your future quality of life will matter more than you can now imagine.

Speaking of hindsight, I still think about that Gibson LG-1. I wonder if it's still there. Maybe I'll head back to the pawn shop in my not-a-Tesla Ford to have a look.

LIGHTS, CAMERAS, ACTION

Okay, Prostate Cancer 101 is over. Now, what are you going to do about *your* prostate cancer?

You know about The Newbie Trap. You can spot the bias and use it to your advantage. You have accepted the unavoidable introduction of risk into your life, and you understand why a decision about your prostate cancer is unavoidable. Timing is tricky, perfection is unlikely, but there are excellent options available today.

Newt is now well-informed, energized, and raring to go. What he needs next is the actionable step-by-step guidance provided in the "9-Step Newbie-Do List" he will find just a few pages from here.

But hold on for just one more minute ...

Fully focus on the next sentence. Chew on it, swallow it, and digest it before you decide how to address your prostate cancer.

The decision is yours alone.

"Of course it is! This is perfectly obvious," says Newt. "Tell me something I don't already know."

Even though we discussed this in the section on bias, I fear that Newt still might not be fully prepared for the tsunami of opinions headed his way. Maybe this has already begun, but the closer he is to a decision, the more intense it could become. Whatever he decides, some people will agree while others will disagree. Some will do so silently while others will be quite vocal and maybe even a little pushy.

As decision-time draws nearer we often tend to become more vulnerable and more easily influenced. The danger is that a "decision" could become little more than acquiescence to the most recent, most vocal, most convincing helpful-minded friend. So, if you experience a lot of flip-flopping, take note. This is serious business, and you cannot afford to join the decision-of-the-day club.

Once you have made a well-considered decision, it should stand. But also remember that it is not wrong to change your mind. It is only wrong to change your mind too often, depending upon which way the wind is blowing. If you are flip-flopping frequently, ask yourself whether you are deliberately making decisions at all, or just going with the flow of the most recent or most forceful input from others.

Remember, you can thank them each for their input without relinquishing your responsibility to decide.

"That's it? Just thank everyone for their input? I feel like there's something else I need from them."

Newt has raised an important point. If you are willing to be a little assertive, you can explicitly tell people what kind of help you do need. Wouldn't it be nice to have a non-judgmental listener who will calmly hear how you feel? Or a sage sounding-board to check your reasoning? How about an interesting conversationalist who can talk about anything but cancer and maybe make you laugh, giving you a much-needed break from the topic? You can help them help you by letting them know what kind of help you want. If you don't, how would they know?

The Rolling Stones said it best: "You can't always get what you want, but if you try sometimes, you just might find you get what you need. Ah, yeah." Wise men, Mick Jagger and Keith Richards. Who knew.

You have gained a ton of insight and it's time to put it to use. Time to take action.

Lights. Cameras.

YOUR 9-STEP NEWBIE-DO LIST

Fasten your seatbelt. Time to get moving. Time for action.

We have explored The Newbie Trap, bias, risk, timing, decisions, perfection, perspective, and more. The net result will have given you a clear-thinking approach to interpreting and understanding the realities of your new situation. It is uncharted territory for most, and a new playbook is required.

So now let's focus on the playbook, on *action*. It is time to take inventory of your situation, put it all together, and do something instead of merely preparing to do something. You are approaching the finish line, and with a little more help and a gentle nudge or two, you will reach it just like I did along with thousands of others. We will review and reassemble the preceding insights and information into an action plan. Newt's Newbie-Do List. *Your* list.

This is your playbook: nine steps, plus a few reminders.

#1: Re-assess your team.

You probably have a primary physician, a urologist, an oncologist, and other highly trained professionals who routinely provide invaluable medical advice. You may also have non-medical specialists who guide you in matters concerning insurance coverage, employment policies, financial planning, and other complex areas. There are likely still others you turn to for personal advice, religious guidance, or psychological-philosophical insight, especially in situations that are challenging. Collectively, these people are your team of advisors, and each of them will play an important role as you move forward.

How long has it been since you honestly reexamined how you feel about each of these essential advisors? Although you may have a high confidence level about the advice you receive from most, there may be one or two with whom you are not as comfortable as you would like to be. Regardless of your history with them, the length of your past association, or their professional stature, you are the final judge of whether they can be helpful in your present situation. If any do not have your full trust and confidence, your decision-making process may be compromised as you attempt to move forward.

In the earlier section on bias, we discussed two tipoffs that are often good reasons to make a change. First is the *my way or the highway* attitude. The other is the excessive use of absolutes, the *always/never* syndrome. If you encounter either of these, watch out and be wary.

Another red flag is lack of access. If getting in touch with someone on your team is an impossible mission, they cannot be of much help. I personally know one doctor who routinely gives his patients his private cell phone number. This is rare, and I asked him why he does it. He had a simple, quick answer. He does it because it is what he would want if the shoe were on the other foot. Furthermore, he added, his patients do not abuse it. Just the opposite. They are respectful and rarely call him. But the peace of mind and reassurance the number provides is huge. Did I mention that he's not just a good doctor, but also a super nice guy?

You cannot make this journey without knowledgeable, trustworthy people to help you evaluate and compare your medical, insurance, employment, and financial options. At times, it can be overwhelming, and you will need competent, supportive, compassionate, accessible people.

This is *your* team. You will not have the time, energy or inclination for second-guessing critical advice as you travel the road ahead. It is not your job to take care of them; it is their role to advise and support *you* during the challenges ahead.

If you need to make changes, do it.

TAKE ACTION: Re-assess your team.

Make sure you feel comfortable with each person on your team of advisors.

If any has not earned your trust, seek other advice in that area.

#2: Answer 5 crucial questions.

The general question, a big one, is easy to ask, harder to answer:

What's your situation?

There has been a lot of information flying around, and Newt is having trouble boiling it down to something manageable. To do this, we'll break it down into five specific questions to help Newt intelligently research and weigh his options, and then make the necessary decisions.

To save Newt from drowning in detail and feeling lost, these Q&As are an intentional oversimplification, not preparation to pass the medical exam. With this in mind, I have kept the discussions ultra-brief, while acknowledging that an entire chapter or book could be devoted to each question. Brevity will make it easier for Newt to periodically review and refocus on the key aspects of his situation.

Newt's urologist or oncologist can help with these questions, but the answers are not always absolute and can involve some degree of subjective interpretation. Because of this, a second opinion may produce additional insight without necessarily negating the first opinion. Feelings should not be hurt if you decide to seek input from more than one source, and if offense is taken, pursuing a second opinion is even more justified.

As a case in point, I recall a guy whose initial Gleason score was 6, as per his urologist. But when the treatment facility evaluated the same biopsy slide, they saw it as a Gleason 7. The slide was then sent to another institute for evaluation, and their interpretation was Gleason 8. To have assumed 6 might have led to a less than optimal treatment plan. This is not to say we all need three sets of eyes on our slide. We typically don't unless there is a specific reason to question it, but it pays to be aware of the subjective nature of some things, and to consider a second opinion when appropriate.

In answering these questions, the specific metrics used (PSA, staging, Gleason score, etc.) can vary, and there will be new and ever-improving diagnostic tools developed over time. However, the questions will remain much the same regardless of which metrics and tools are used at the time of your diagnosis.

Here are the questions, in no particular order:

- **Was it caught early?** Intermediate? Advanced? This is generally identified by one of four **staging** categories, with stage T1 as earliest, stage T4 as most advanced. Staging is more complex than merely a T1 to T4 scale, but this is a good place to start developing your big picture. Your **PSA** history and current level are also indicators, with lower or slowly rising scores often indicating early diagnosis.
- **Is it fully contained** within the prostate, or were cancerous cells found outside the prostate, too? The T1-T4 staging metric also helps with this: T1 and T2 cancers are likely contained within the prostate, and T3-T4 cancers are likely to have spread beyond it. Additional diagnostics are sometimes needed.
- **Is it aggressive?** A **Gleason** score of 6 is not usually regarded as aggressive, 7 is moderately so, and above that is most aggressive. As I described above, you should not be surprised if the interpretation of your biopsy samples varies. Another indicator of aggressiveness is the rate at which the **PSA** has been rising, with a quickly rising PSA being more aggressive.
- **Do you have any symptoms?** Prostate cancer, especially when caught early, often has no symptoms. If you do have prostate-cancer-like symptoms, they are not to be ignored. They might relate to your cancer or to another condition with similar symptoms. Either way, you need to know, and they should always be disclosed.
- **How healthy are you**, other than having prostate cancer? How are you currently functioning in terms of urination, defecation, and sexual function? How old are you now? Before your cancer diagnosis, how many more years were you reasonably hoping to live? Every one of us will eventually reach the end of our road, and the amount of anticipated travel time remaining can influence what you do about your cancer.

Gleaning a good sense of your cancer-related circumstances—*your situation*—can be as challenging as researching treatments. When you and Newt can answer these five questions with a reasonable level of confidence, you will have a pretty good handle on your situation and will be ready to intelligently move forward.

Keep your answers in mind as you consider options. They are *your* options to treat *your* prostate cancer in *your* body in *your* life. For any therapy, the question is not merely whether it is a good one, but whether it is a good one *for you,* in light of your unique set of circumstances. One size does not fit all.

What's *your* situation?

> **TAKE ACTION: Answer 5 crucial questions.**
>
> Review and clarify your answers to these questions:
>
> Was it caught early? Is it fully contained? Is it aggressive? Are you symptomatic? How is your general health?

#3: Identify your tolerance for risk.

By now, Newt is well aware of the prostate cancer therapy tradeoff, and there is no way to sugarcoat it. We all have to face it, and so does Newt. We can either defer treatment and risk allowing the cancer to progress, or treat it and risk allowing unpleasant side effects to become part of our life. We can hope to avoid both, but there is no guaranteed path for doing so. Most of us ultimately seek a therapy we believe is most likely to control or cure our cancer with minimal or no side effects. This is what I did, and so far (*10 Years After*) it has worked out well.

In 2010 I believed that proton therapy would give me the best chance of achieving both objectives, with the least risk of failing at either. On one hand, it felt a little like a random roll of the dice—as would any therapy—but it also simultaneously seemed like a relatively safe and sound approach, not as risky as other choices. If I had viewed proton as an exciting, ultra-new, highly promising technology on the bleeding edge, I would not have done it. Too risky for conservative ol' me. But based on science that made intuitive sense to me, and with a successful track record of more than a quarter century, it was a good fit for my cautious low-risk nature.

But that's me, and Newt is Newt, and you are you. Are you more comfortable with greater risk than I am? I will not stand near the edge of the roof of a parking garage, even when there is a chest-high wall or a sturdy rail. My brain shuts down the effort after determining there is nothing to gain and a lot to lose by standing too close to the edge. *Ron, back away from the edge. Awaaaaaay from the edge!*

Where would you stand? Are you a natural risk-taker, ready to put the pedal to the metal with aggressive or new approaches? Or like me, are you more comfortable with a cautious, conservative, measured consideration of well-established therapies with a track record? Do you maintain a speed of no more than four miles per hour over the limit, or do you push it to nine, or even more? Are you more inclined to avoid a ticket and safely reach your destination soon enough, or to accept a greater risk of a ticket or accident hoping to arrive a little earlier?

If you are in the latter group, then be bold. Search for clinical trials or innovative technologies and at least consider any new therapies you are hopeful about. Just remember that this approach is called "cutting edge," or maybe even "bleeding edge," for a reason. Although it has a big potential payoff, it is correspondingly more uncertain. Nevertheless, if you are a *pedal to the metal* kind of guy, this is absolutely a legitimate approach.

To test whether you genuinely fall into this cutting-edge group, close your eyes and imagine that you have completed any of the current mainstream treatments and achieved a reasonably good, but not perfect outcome. You are sitting at the kitchen table with your best friend, sipping your massive morning cups of coffee, talking about life.

Now imagine this conversation:

Friend: You know, I still think about how worried I was when you had that nasty cancer thing happen a while ago. Close call. Dodged that bullet, thank goodness. I have precious few friends and can't afford to lose any, not even you!

You: Gee, thanks. Yeah, dodged that bullet, but now I have this other little thing to deal with. I told you about it. Not horrible, but really annoying. I guess I can handle it.

Friend: Well, sorry about that, but here we are, enjoying the morning, shooting the breeze, just like always.

You: Sure, but a day doesn't go by when I don't wish I had taken a chance on that new therapy like Jack did. He's cancer-free, and no side effects. None! And he knows two other guys who did it. I should have done *that*. Oh well. Shoulda woulda coulda, right?

Does that exchange seem realistic? Does it feel like it fits you? Are you saying, *yep, that would be me*? If so, then now is your chance to be bold, provided that you can accept the riskier nature of Jack's approach and won't later berate yourself for not having taken a more conventional path, no matter what happens. Because the flipside of this conversation could be this:

Friend: You know, I still think about how worried I was when you had that nasty cancer thing happen a while ago. Close call. Dodged that bullet, thank goodness. I have precious few friends and can't afford to lose any, not even you!

You: Gee, thanks. Yeah, dodged that bullet, but now I have this other little thing to deal with. I told you about it. Not horrible, but really annoying. I guess I can handle it.

Friend: Well, sorry about that, but here we are, enjoying the morning, shooting the breeze, just like always.

You: Sure, but a day doesn't go by when I don't wish I had done something normal instead of taking a chance on that stupid new therapy that left me with this nasty little problem. You know, Jack took the usual route like most people, and he got rid of his cancer with no side effects. None! And he knows two other guys who did the same thing, same result. I should have done that. Oh well. Shoulda woulda coulda, right?

If you can decide now which conversation is a better fit for your possible future, you will have a good idea of where you stand on the risk-taking spectrum. Also remember that in either example, you might be the other guy, Jack, who cured his cancer with no side effects. For him, these conversations need never happen. He might not think about any of this again at all. If you, like me, are as fortunate as Jack, then this entire exercise will ultimately become a moot point. If only you could see into the future. Darn.

You can also gain insight into your risk-taking profile by examining other areas of your life, unrelated to cancer. Your reaction during past events can be illuminating. Although you may not have thought about it in these terms, your risk profile might already be well-established and ingrained. Mine is, and in some situations it kicks in automatically, as in the parking garage roof example above, and also at the theater.

I recall purchasing excellent front row balcony tickets for a play my wife and I were eager to see. I can still picture climbing the stairs and beginning the final trek to our center seats. The chairs were to my right, and to my left was what my cerebral command control center identified as a totally inadequate risky rail, a modest barrier to my probable death. Involuntarily, my knees instantly buckled, dropping me down to a safe stance completely below the rail, leaving Lucy looking around wondering how I had suddenly disappeared. On hands and knees I then crawled to my seat, climbed in, clenched the armrests, and enjoyed the play.

I should note that I was the only one crawling to his seat. Apparently, nobody else felt at risk walking upright along the rail. Perception of risk is a personal matter, and yours is the only one that matters. In 2010, despite its long, successful track record, proton therapy was regarded as risky or experimental by some, but not by me and many others. Today, there is ongoing debate about when or whether active surveillance can be a good bet with early diagnosis, but likewise, what matters is each man's perspective.

The bottom line is that understanding your tolerance for risk now will help lead you to choices you can most comfortably live with later. Think about it now, not later, and be honest about it.

Newt will require some serious introspection, and he will need to be careful. He might mistakenly ask what his risk profile *should* be, rather than what it really is. We each have a natural comfort level concerning risk, and it is important to truthfully identify and embrace yours. To pretend it is otherwise or to disregard it can leave you less likely to choose a plan you can live with without regret.

As with most choices in life, acceptance of more risk opens the possibility for greater reward, but also for greater loss. It's the nature of the beast. We have no trouble grasping this in financial terms; indeed, identifying your risk profile is one of the first tasks most investment advisors will require. Health professionals may not be as direct, but your risk profile is extremely relevant in medical matters, too.

The prostate cancer tradeoff, absolute cure versus zero side effects, influenced my choice, and will almost certainly be a factor for you, too. Be bold or be conservative. But be honest.

I no longer buy tickets for front-row balcony seats.

> **TAKE ACTION: Identify your tolerance for risk.**
>
> To avoid regrets later,
> honestly identify and embrace your risk profile now.
> Are you most comfortable with cutting edge or tried-and-true?

#4: Consider your mind along with your body.

Most of us focus heavily on predicting the possible physical results of the treatment choices we make, but we often forget to pay attention to our future psychological well-being. Anticipating how you will feel later as a result of decisions you make today is as important as it is difficult. Knowing and embracing your tolerance for risk is part of the picture, but there is more.

A friend of mine, slightly older than me, had prostate cancer before I did. He had no difficulty figuring out what to do. For him, there was little if any research into current technology, no past patient interviews, no investigation of cancer centers nationwide.

Just one overriding psychological imperative: *Get. It. Out.* He had a visceral disgust with the idea that cancer was in his body, in his prostate. Surgery was the only way to satisfy his need to cleanse his body of the intrusion, and I applaud him for recognizing this and doing what he had to do.

His decision was based on sanity. He instinctively knew that for his future peace of mind, removing the prostate was the only option. Fortunately, things have gone well for him. Most importantly, he seems happy and is clearly enjoying every day of his life.

For me, it was the opposite. I had a visceral reaction to the idea of a blade slicing into me to cut out and remove my prostate. I was similarly uncomfortable with radioactive seeds being placed permanently in my prostate, so brachytherapy was undesirable. I was eager to find an alternative and more than willing to do the research. Once I learned about proton therapy, I knew it fit the bill as an effective, non-invasive option that suited me nicely.

My friend and I have good lives, with no regrets about our personal choices for cancer treatment. To each their own. Different strokes for different folks. And most importantly, it pays to know thyself. Three possibly overused platitudes that are popular for good reason and apply here perfectly.

Maybe you are philosophically or religiously against any "unnatural" intervention including surgery, radiation, chemotherapy, and others. Rather than compromise your beliefs and feel hypocritical for life, you may want to try a more holistic approach involving nutrition, exercise, meditation, and other techniques you perceive to be more natural. If you are willing to accept the results of this controversial approach whatever the outcome, and if you can tolerate the inevitable criticism, then you have found your comfort zone.

Making your final decision about how to proceed based solely on considerations like those above might not be a great idea, but you should include them in the mix. If your feelings are strong, you would be unwise to ignore them. Your feelings about whatever you do will have an impact on your mind, just as any treatment you choose will have an impact on your body. Both are important, and neither should be overlooked or ignored. Your challenge is to find a healthy balance between them because your future feelings and frame of mind will have a huge influence on your quality of life.

There is no universal "right" or "wrong" about it, so be totally honest with yourself, try to imagine your future self, and make your best educated guess at how you will react to the treatment you are considering.

> **TAKE ACTION: Consider your mind along with your body.**
>
> As you naturally focus on the physical side of things, remember that the emotional impact matters, too.

#5: Do your research (due diligence).

Newt is making progress. He has a good team. He understands the key aspects of his situation. And he has a good handle on his tolerance for risk. He is now ready to do some serious research.

Or is he?

Newt might be more of a seat-of-the-pants gut reaction kind of decisionmaker than a researcher, which is fine. Or he might be most comfortable simply going along with the recommendation of a trusted friend, doctor, or past patient, also fine. If either approach is genuinely Newt's style of decision-making, there is no need for him to do due diligence. Of course, the decision and responsibility would nevertheless remain Newt's, even if his choices are based on his instinct or an advisor.

But I happen to know Newt quite well, and neither of these approaches is his. He's more like me. He digs for data and he asks a lot of questions. Newt is definitely ready to dive into the deep end of his research, his due diligence. He is eager to reach an acceptable level of knowledge and confidence with an answer to the looming question:

"What are my options, and which one is best for me?"

Newt needs to find reliable information about today's treatment options, the likelihood of success for each, and the associated risks. It's a big job, and neither books nor any single type of resource can provide all the information he will need. Medical websites and publications, conversations with doctors, anecdotal stories from patients (see: "The Newbie Trap"), online prostate cancer groups, information from cancer treatment centers, and yes, even books can provide useful information, but none alone is sufficient. As I said, it's a big job.

In previous sections I addressed many issues relating to research, but I have a few more tips to share with Newt. He needs no help finding information. He knows how to do that quite well, and in today's world it is not particularly difficult. The challenging part is knowing what to do with the massive amount of data that is there for the taking. Harder yet is to know when to stop researching, and to recognize the writing on the wall once it becomes visible.

Dealing with cancer is a journey, and doing the research is a journey of its own. Answers will develop like old Polaroid photographs, not instantly, nor as a sudden aha moment. Instead, you will inevitably notice emerging patterns that will gradually coalesce, leading us to develop greater confidence about some avenues and less about others. You won't find the single "right" answer, nor a perfect solution. There is none. The mission is to reach a sufficient level of confidence about an approach that feels right.

Sufficient, not necessarily 100%.

Then, when your research seems to be pointing in one direction, become your own devil's advocate. When you are beginning to feel good about an option, try to find negatives about it. A relative lack of negatives will give you even greater confidence in your positive feeling.

However, while you certainly should explore the negatives, keep in mind that everything has its share of complainers, and unhappy chronic contrarians often tend to be louder than satisfied supporters. No siree, there will be no shortage of critics for any option. While some may offer legitimate critical information, others will be little more than compulsive whiners, so take them with a grain of salt. However, if you find a recurring theme in the critical reviews, it is more likely to be a legitimate concern worth investigating further. Finally, always consider any criticism in the larger context of everything you have learned so you can decide objectively whether it may be valid.

An important caveat about cost: Save yourself a lot of time and distraction by resisting the natural temptation to research costs as you investigate therapies. To be sure, costs may ultimately be a limiting factor, but determining this should be the second step after you have first listed and ranked your preferred therapies. Finding a reasonably accurate estimate of your out-of-pocket cost for any treatment is complicated, if not impossible for you, and trying to do so will drain time and energy better spent on evaluating options for treatment. You can defer the important question of money until later. Cost estimation should not be part of due diligence, nor used to prematurely eliminate any options. [See Newbie-Do step #8 for more about the matter of cost.]

One last tip, and maybe the most important one. As you perform your due diligence, take occasional breaks to live your life. Have a beer, or at least a Diet Coke. Read a good book or go to the movies. Play some pickleball or take a walk. Do something fun with someone you love. When you resume researching, this will help you remember why you're doing it.

> **TAKE ACTION: Do your research.**
>
> Explore all available types of information sources. Watch for emerging patterns that will lead you toward an option you feel confident about.

#6: Commit to a plan.

Make a decision.
Research may be fun and rewarding, but it is not your goal; it is a means toward *achieving* your goal of making a reasonable decision about how best to proceed. But your first decision, a difficult one, is to end the research, because unless you make a proactive decision to do so, you will have decided to accept the default of watchful waiting. Either way, it's a decision. Until you decide to do something else, you will have decided to wait, and filling the time with more research doesn't change this.

Somewhat ironically, it is the waiting—you can call it researching if you prefer—that can make you increasingly anxious. While in this mode, you might fret over the anticipation that your anxiety will worsen once you commit to a treatment plan, a worry which can add to your decision avoidance. It is a fear of commitment.

Believe me when I tell you that the opposite is more likely. Once you declare an end to your research and move forward with a plan, there is often a great sense of relief. If you are expecting increased anxiety, this relief will come as a pleasant surprise. You will have jettisoned the stressful burden of making a decision and replaced it with a plan, a timeline, and a target. Light at the end of the tunnel. Ahhhh, yes! Feels good, doesn't it!

I have seen this time after time. It is no longer a surprise when a man on the verge of a decision calls me for a final nudge. He will say something like, "I'm about 95% ready to go with proton." Not being one to push, I might ask, "What's holding you back? What do you need to hit 100% and get moving?" Nearly every time his response will be, "I guess nothing is really holding me back, and I have pretty much decided to go with proton, but gee, I don't know, I'm just not sure."

Yes he is. He's sure. He may also be afraid of making a mistake, but he is nevertheless sure. I often receive a follow-up communication thanking me for helping him decide, but all I did was ask a question. He did the work, and he was clearly already there. I guess you could call that a nudge, just a tiny poke to urge him over the line he had already decided to cross.

No one will impose a due date for this assignment. It's up to you, so do a reasonable amount of research. Then commit to a plan of action and move forward. You will have all the time in the world to engage in fun, exciting, endless research later, after you have cured your cancer. But now, draw your line in the sand, take your best shot, and do something.

> **TAKE ACTION: Commit to a plan.**
> As soon as your confidence level is sufficiently high, make a decision and commit to a plan.
> You cannot research forever.

#7: Apply for treatment.

Now the fun begins.

If your decision was to engage in active surveillance, you can bookmark this page and return later, if and when you have decided to pursue treatment. Otherwise, clap your hands once loudly, say "Here we go!" with conviction, and then get cracking! Schedule the procedure or apply to one or more facilities offering the type of treatment you chose. For some procedures, you need to do little more than schedule an appointment following a doctor's referral. For others, you can often submit your initial application online, or you can request an application by phone.

There is no reason to delay applying. There is no fee, no commitment, nothing to lose, and you can bail out at any point for any reason. On the other hand, you can learn a lot by starting the application process, possibly including an initial consultation and maybe some further diagnostic tests. If a particular center does not satisfy your criteria or if you do not meet their qualifications, wouldn't you like to know sooner than later? Of course, they might be a perfect match, and if so, wouldn't you like to find out?

Many men, including Newt, apply to more than one facility, which is fine. I did not. I approached it the same way I approached college, much to the displeasure of my high school advisor. I wanted to attend the University of Michigan, assumed they would take me, and applied only there. This drove my advisor nearly insane because he was adamant that everyone, including me, needed a backup. But I paid him no heed, U. of M. took me (Go Blue!), and that was that. I admit it was not necessarily the best strategy, but I was lucky and it worked out well.

Old habits die hard. More than four decades later I was sure I wanted proton therapy at the University of Florida Health Proton Therapy Institute in Jacksonville. I did request information from a few non-proton centers who sent me their promo material, which only reinforced my original inclination. I applied only to UF Proton and just weeks later I was on the slab getting the beam (i.e., on the treatment table receiving proton therapy). So like college, I applied, I got in, and the rest is history.

If you have already determined that a particular facility is where you want to receive treatment, you can apply only there, following my approach. If there are several facilities you are considering, you can apply to them all at once, like Newt. An application is not a commitment to be treated. Rather, it is an invitation for a facility to convince you to choose them over the alternatives. It is an opportunity for them to put their best foot forward and quickly convey a high level of confidence that they can and will serve you well. Remember, they are a business and you are the customer.

An application is a two-way street: you must accept them, and they must accept you.

Your first point of contact will typically be someone in the intake department, and your contact person should respond expeditiously. It is perfectly reasonable to expect the application packet to arrive the next business day. Cancer is urgent, and their response should demonstrate that they understand and respect this. If your contact cannot be reached easily or does not respond quickly or appropriately at this early stage of your relationship, why should you trust that the rest of their process will be better? Your first contact should give you confidence as well as comfort. You should expect no less from the organization you hope to entrust with your care and your life.

Likewise, if you have scheduled a procedure based on a doctor's referral, you should expect quick, complete, and easily understandable instructions that prepare you for precisely what to do and expect before, during, and afterward. It should be clear how to contact someone if you have questions. Your confidence should rightfully be affected by the level of personal attention and accessibility demonstrated by those involved in the procedure. It is their job to make the process clear. If you are confused, it is not your fault. Reach out and let someone know you need clarification.

If your concerns are more than just the natural butterflies in your stomach felt before any treatment begins, you can always cancel a procedure for any reason at any time, even the day before. This may seem extreme and possibly unfair, but I know several men who did just that. They had never been told about proton therapy and were well on their way to a radical prostatectomy. Then, just days before surgery, they learned about proton and decided it was a better option for them. Despite the short notice, they canceled their surgery and shifted gears. With new information, you have the right and responsibility to use it rather than ignore it, even if it puts you on an entirely new path, regardless of any regrettable inconvenience it might cause.

The information in an application packet should answer most of your main questions, including how to obtain answers not addressed in the standard packet. I ask a lot of questions. They just pop into my head and I ask, sometimes to the displeasure of those who must answer. I'm not sure if there is a name for my question-asking disorder, but there should be. Excessive Question Asking Syndrome? It is an affliction, albeit an often useful one. In case your mind does not work in a similar manner, allow me to provide some questions to get you started.

How soon will they be able to schedule your treatment? Are there medical procedures to complete before they can consider you for treatment? Are there any pre-treatment restrictions in your diet or activity? How much help can they provide with financial and insurance issues? Who will be your primary contact or case manager? Who will be your contact for financial matters? How can you quickly reach them? What is the exact nature of the financial commitment they require? How will you be expected to handle out-of-pocket fees? Will they submit the necessary insurance paperwork for you and obtain the authorizations required? If the facility is out of town, will they provide housing advice? What will be expected of you once treatment is complete? What kind of follow-up relationship will they have with you after treatment? If they are out of town, how closely will they work with your local doctors?

All these questions are reasonable. I expected courteous, complete responses and so should you. It is their job to provide clear answers to your questions, and like me, you will have many, even if yours are not caused by a question-asking disorder. To be fair, we cannot expect everyone to know everything about everything, and not all questions have answers. "I don't know, but I'll help you find out," or "I wish I could tell you, but there simply isn't an answer for that" might be the right answer. Regardless, ask your questions. All of them.

Ultimately, the above steps will result in a mutual acceptance between you and a facility offering the treatment you want. Their personnel will guide you through the steps necessary to reach the finish line.

> **TAKE ACTION: Apply for treatment.**
> Apply at one or more facilities and notice how they respond.
>
> An application is not a commitment,
> any appointment can be canceled,
> and you can shift gears at any time if you lose confidence.
>
> You have cancer.
> You should expect to be treated with all due urgency.

#8: Develop your strategy.

This is where the rubber meets the road. It is where you either go around, through, under, or over any remaining obstacles and put pedal to the metal to reach the finish line.

Yes, there may still be obstacles that are your final challenges on your road to curing cancer: time off from work, insurance issues, out-of-pocket expenses, transportation to and from a facility, and out-of-town housing. Plus, you may need to find someone to water the plants, feed the cat, and take care of your mother-in-law. Yikes.

We fully addressed such issues in our previous discussion of perspective. Here in this "action" section I will repackage that information into a more concise *what-to-do* format. After all, it's your Newbie-Do List, and this item #8 is about addressing anything standing in your way on the road to a cure, especially matters relating to time or money.

If you expect to be unavailable for an extended period while battling cancer, talk with your family, friends, employer, and others affected by your possible absence. They can help you find creative solutions to meet any of your responsibilities that cannot be neglected. It doesn't matter whether they or you initiate the conversation, but make sure the discussion happens so you can take the time to do what's necessary to prepare for your absence.

If you are worried about your job responsibilities while fighting cancer, discuss it with your boss or human resources department. There may well be a way to make it work.

If you are self-employed, will you lose clients? Talk openly to them about it and you may be surprised at the compassion, understanding, and flexibility they will often demonstrate.

If you are someone's primary caregiver, talk with anyone who could potentially pitch in and help while you are unavailable. Even if nobody else could provide care the way you do, someone else can surely give adequate care for a while.

If paying for treatment is a possible issue, remember that your treatment facility can be a great source of experienced help, so ask for it. If you have an accountant or financial advisor, invite them to offer some creative approaches to funding your therapy. Even a local banker you've never met might have some insights into how you can leverage any of the resources you have and might identify resources you overlooked. There's nothing to lose and everything to gain by asking, so ask them all.

Make a list of all your personal and financial resources to reference as you consider using them. Your employer might not be as unreasonable as you fear. Your insurance company might be more likely to approve coverage upon an appeal than they were after your initial request. Your family may be able to help in ways you did not anticipate. Plan A may be more of a possibility than you initially thought.

Also remember that your treatment facility could be your greatest advocate, so let their financial/insurance experts go to bat for you. You're on the same team, and it is in your best interest and theirs to use all the tricks in the book to make it affordable for you to be treated there. This is their job, and they are usually pretty darn good at it. They often know of techniques or opportunities you would never discover on your own. You are not their first patient with financial concerns, so give them a shot at helping you.

Do your absolute best to pursue every available avenue and use every available resource to get what you want, if you truly want it. This is important. What you do now will impact the rest of your life. You have done the research. You have evaluated your options. You have made a decision.

Now make it happen.

TAKE ACTION: Develop your strategy.

You will need many resources and great determination to win your battle with cancer.

You have made a commitment. You have a plan.
Now make it happen.

#9: Focus on the future.

Congratulations. You made it!

You will hopefully be on the road to recovery soon. In most cases, prostate cancer treatments carry a high probability of success, and you have every reason to be optimistic. Much of the hard work in this battle is now behind you. The rest is mostly up to your medical team and support system. The proverbial ball is now rolling.

You made the best decision you could, and as you move forward you should not second-guess yourself. Sure, there may have been other paths you could have followed, but so what? There are no do-overs, and you can't change the past. Why not allow yourself the small pleasure of knowing you did your due diligence and were thorough and methodical in your approach? That part of this adventure is over, and you have earned the right to focus on the future.

Life is never without trials and tribulations. You have had to confront prostate cancer in addition to other challenges you have already faced and some you have yet to encounter. You might feel sorry for yourself and even angry that you have had to deal with cancer, but look around you. It could be much worse, and others are facing hardships much greater than yours. This was certainly true for me.

No one makes it through life without encountering obstacles, and in the scheme of things, prostate cancer is not among the worst. Sure, you might fear having some side effects sooner or later, and you could be a bit wary about having a second bout with cancer. Those feelings are normal and fine, as long as you don't let them prevent you from enjoying life.

Your treatment, and hopefully your cancer, will soon become distant memories, but your life will have changed forever. Other far less traumatic events have changed your life, and it only makes sense that prostate cancer will have a major impact. The good news is that many, maybe even most of the changes will be positive.

It may sound trite, but you will have a renewed appreciation for life, and will be more likely to live each day to its fullest potential. Your new perspective can motivate you to reprioritize. It can help you focus without delay on what matters most to you. You will have new friends who have shared your experience, and you will be in a position to help others facing a similar challenge.

Ironically, you will have gained a lot. I certainly did.

Breathe easy, enjoy your life, and don't look back.

> **TAKE ACTION: Focus on the future.**
>
> Prostate cancer is just one of many challenges in your life.
>
> Appreciate and enjoy the positive changes
> that result from meeting this challenge.
>
> Look ahead, live every day to the fullest, and don't look back.

Okay, there you have it: Your 9-Step Newbie-Do List. I've summarized it for you in a handy checklist format. Complete these action items one by one and you'll be on your way. Yes, you have my permission to write in your book.

- ☐ Re-assess your team.
- ☐ Answer 5 crucial questions.
- ☐ Identify your tolerance for risk.
- ☐ Consider your mind along with your body.
- ☐ Do your research.
- ☐ Commit to a plan.
- ☐ Apply for treatment.
- ☐ Develop your strategy.
- ☐ Focus on the future.

A Private Conversation with Proton Ambassadors

I am a card-carrying proton ambassador. Here is my card:

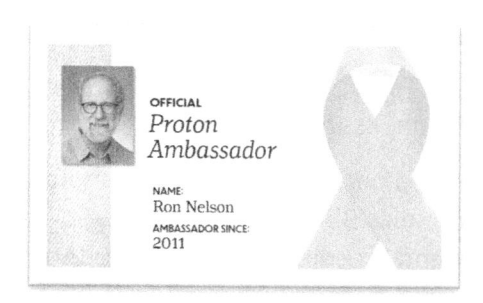

OFFICIAL
Proton Ambassador

NAME:
Ron Nelson
AMBASSADOR SINCE:
2011

    I am also an author, a blogger, and a speaker on the topics of prostate cancer and proton therapy. Yet, I hesitate to recommend proton therapy. Before you jump to any conclusions, please allow me to explain.

    I am relentlessly contacted, as I suspect you are, too, by companies I have recently dealt with, asking me whether I would recommend them—a question I take seriously and literally. My bank, credit card company, hardware store, online merchant, coffee roastery, airline, restaurant, and even the guy who sold me a package of four #10 x ¾" Phillips flat head wood screws. They all want my endorsement expressed as a numeric rating of the likelihood I would recommend them, their product, or their service.

    They are not asking whether I am satisfied, which is a very different question. They are asking whether I would recommend them, and I am not sure what their exact intention is with this solicitation. Are they asking whether I wander about, randomly tapping people on the shoulder, touting their offering?

Me, to a random passerby:
> Hey, buddy, sorry to interrupt, but you really ought to fly on Super-Duper Airways, which I highly recommend! I can also suggest an awesome toaster, if you want!

Random passerby:
> ???????????????????

Or are they asking whether I lie in wait, perpetually ready to pounce, watching for any excuse to toot their horn?

Jane: You know, Ron, I sure am hungry.

Ron: Hey, I have the perfect solution! You should head right over to Hungry Hank's BBQ Pit and top off your tank! That's what I did once, and I recommend you do it, too!

So no, even if I am an extremely satisfied customer, I am unlikely to be a proactive promoter. As a matter of course, I simply do not make a habit of approaching people to offer my opinion about random things I love. I would regard such an interaction as weird and inappropriate, regardless of which side of the conversation I found myself on.

Of course, if I were *asked* for an opinion then it would be a different matter. But I am rarely asked to make such recommendations, so I don't. None of the survey questions specify "if asked," and the likelihood of an unsolicited spontaneous and intrusive recommendation from me is near zero, which would have to be my honest survey response. But the goose-egg rating would be misleading because I do like my bank, my restaurant, and yes, even my toaster. And if you ask, I will enthusiastically tell you all you want to know. Maybe more.

Nor will I tackle unsuspecting strangers or friends to ask if they know about proton therapy and how amazing it is, blasting the tumor while radiating much less healthy tissue than conventional radiation does. I just don't do that unless asked.

Okay, maybe I do, sometimes, just a little.

In any case, I am extremely careful about how I portray myself as a proton ambassador, as I hope you are, too. Although we are just regular guys who were once newbies and are now proton alumni trying to be helpful, we have been endowed with authority and must behave accordingly. Our words can significantly impact the lives of others and must be chosen with sensitivity and purpose.

Even when a prostate cancer newbie specifically asks me if I recommend proton therapy, I hesitate. I am not a doctor, he is not my patient, and I know little about his medical situation or history. I carefully avoid making medical recommendations, and because I realize the weight of my words, I do not recommend proton or any other therapy to him.

But I *do* strongly recommend that he *consider* proton therapy. Yes, absolutely consider it.

I recognize that you may view these distinctions as petty, picky, trivial semantic distinctions—using "recommend *considering* proton therapy" instead of simply saying "recommend proton therapy," or caring whether or not "if asked" is specified, and so on. But words matter. Our interpretation of the words used by others, and the ones we choose to represent our own position—all of these words can impact the life of a newbie, and we must choose them carefully.

If we recognize our power to influence the life-changing decisions a newbie must make, then it is incumbent upon us to wield it responsibly. Toward that end, I will share my insights about being a better, more effective advocate of proton therapy, including some surprising hidden nuance that affects our interactions as proton ambassadors.

MY STATUS AS A PROTON AMBASSADOR

I have had some animated interactions with my wife Lucy debating my status as an ambassador for proton therapy. Am I one, or not? If I am one, what kind of proton ambassador am I?

Ron: I do think proton is great, but I'm not exactly a flag-waving ambassador. I never tell anyone they should have proton therapy, I never spontaneously recommend proton therapy, and I am not a member of any pro-proton organizations. What kind of ambassador is *that*?

Lucy: Ron, don't be ridiculous! You absolutely *are* a proton ambassador. You speak publicly about proton, you write about it, and you explain its benefits to anyone who will listen, and even to some who would rather not. And I have seen you spend endless time talking with newbies who contact you to ask questions about proton therapy. If that doesn't make you an ambassador, what would?

Yes, folks, that is the question. What precisely must we do as proton ambassadors? Do I qualify, and do you? Like me, you supposedly are one, or at least might become one, so it seems like a good idea to explore what exactly an ambassador is, and what it takes to be a good one. Surely, we ought to know what we signed up for and how to do it well.

A definition would help us, and I was tempted to quote some dictionary definitions. My first draft included a pretty good one from the Cambridge Dictionary. But my editor (a.k.a., wife) tossed it out, claiming that the technique of citing dictionary definitions is very high-school-paper-ish. Well. I'm no longer in high school, so I guess I'm on my own.

Or preferably, as the title of this chapter implies, we can make it a conversation and explore this together. Being labeled *ambassador* has implications, and we ambassadors should discuss it among ourselves. What does the term imply about us? More importantly, what *should* we be as proton ambassadors?

I will share my point of view here, and you can respond with yours (Ron@AfterProton.com). I hope you will, because I am sure you have additional insights that are valuable and can help *me* become a better proton ambassador. I thank you in advance.

Now back to the question. What is an ambassador?

THE SELF-APPOINTED AMBASSADOR

To explore this, I'll use another pretend person to represent anyone on the Ambassador List for the fictitious ZapMe Proton Center. I'll call him Al, short for **A**mbassador **L**ist. Al's job as an ambassador is ostensibly to help Newt, the fictitious newbie-in-need in our proton fantasyland. Newt was created in the "For Newbies Only" section, which you may have skipped if you're an ambassador, not a newbie.

Al is a self-appointed authority on proton therapy and possibly also prostate cancer. And we know that his audience of newbies does indeed regard him as an authority of sorts. Otherwise, why would they care what he has to say? Clearly, they believe he has good, valid information, and they value his input.

However, in all but rare cases Al's only qualification is being a former patient. To put it more crudely, he was one of ZapMe's customers, and that's it. Based only on this, designating him as an authority on proton therapy seems a bit like considering me to be a knowledgeable auto mechanic because I have driven a car, or a talented film director because I have gone to the movies. Makes no sense.

On the other hand, I can certainly test drive a car and offer a valid opinion from a driver's point of view. I could be a movie critic (and I am), although I'm not sure anyone would care to hear what I think about Star Wars (I'm a Trekkie) or any movie. Then again, Newbies do seek Al's opinions. And when all is said and done, that's all that matters. I can be a movie critic if someone cares to listen, and similarly, Al can be a proton ambassador if anyone wants his input. And so he is.

How does ZapMe feel about it? Do they want Al to have this role? Of course they do, but with a major caveat. ZapMe must be ultra-careful to avoid giving even the accidental appearance of endorsing Al or any individual to speak officially on their behalf. They cannot control what Al or the many others like him might say, how they say it, or to whom. Al, even with the best of intentions, is completely untrained, unfiltered, answers to nobody, and might quite innocently say just the wrong thing in the wrong place at the wrong time. This would represent a huge liability risk for ZapMe, possibly also involving potential HIPAA violations with serious consequences. ZapMe is therefore crystal clear in stating that Al does not represent them in any official capacity, even while being thrilled that he is a cheerleader for them and proton.

Nevertheless, even as a free agent with no formal status, Al is one of ZapMe's most effective marketing resources. Satisfied and vocal customers like Al are invaluable because on a peer-to-peer basis, they are highly trusted. Al may not be part of the official marketing organization, the paid professionals employed by ZapMe, but his value cannot be overstated. Priceless, as they say.

Al's unofficial status is not only with respect to ZapMe. He also does not officially represent or speak for his own group of people—men with prostate cancer, or even men treated at ZapMe. That is, unless he leads a support group or has some other official role in the prostate cancer community. But regardless, all of us in this huge club-nobody-wants-to-join, do sort of represent each other. Whether or not we actively promote our favorite therapy, anyone close to us who encounters prostate cancer will seek our advice. Because we have walked the walk, we are presumed to be knowledgeable about the road we travel. And newbies will naturally turn to us for help as they venture forth into the unknown.

Where does that leave us? As a proton ambassador, what exactly is Al's role, and what should it be?

WHAT NEWBIES WANT FROM AMBASSADORS

In defining Al's role as an ambassador, we can frame the question in two ways, from two surprisingly different points of view. We can ask what newbies want from Al, or we can ask what Al seeks to accomplish. On the surface, we might expect these to match, but as we dig a little deeper we will learn this is not always the case.

So first let's ask, what does a newbie like Newt want from Al? To repeat the answer from the previous chapter, *a newbie's overriding objective is to clear the fog and find the road back to his pre-cancer "normal" life ASAP.* Newt wants Al to help him accomplish this. No small feat.

Let's peel back the layers of Newt's pre-cancer life. He had no reason yet to suspect he might have prostate cancer, and probably rarely if ever thought about the disease, despite its prevalence. It is no surprise that he does not want to think about it today, or ever again. As a newbie, Newt wants Al to help reveal a roadmap to the total erasure of prostate cancer from his mind and his future. He does not yet know that it will likely become a permanent influence in his life. Only later will he realize that even if completely cured, he may continue to be at least a little wary of a possible recurrence or side effects.

Peeling to the next layer, Newt was never as anxious about his future as he is now. He is embarking on a journey into the unknown, and not knowing what his future holds can be nerve-wracking. Newt wants the kind of normal-ish life Al appears to be living, free of cancer-related stress and anxiety. Whatever the stress-relieving trick may be, he wants Al to share the magic.

Related to the stress, Newt wants reassurance. A newbie can find it difficult to envision a world in which everything is okay again. Al seems to live in that world, and just by seeing him, Newt can gain confidence that he, too, will be okay. Maybe Al can offer some information to help make that happen.

Removing cancer from the radar, or at least reducing stress and anxiety while gaining hope—these are the results Newt wants, but probably mostly on a subconscious level. On a more imminent and practical level, Newt's objective is obvious: He wants Al to guide him implicitly by example, or by outlining the next steps. Where should he go? Who should he call? What should he say? How should he deal with the timing, the cost, the logistics?

What should he do to make everything right again? This is the giant-of-a-question underlying Newt's entire reason for contacting ambassadors. Once he has made a firm decision, he will rarely contact anyone else on the list of proton ambassadors. He will be putting all his energy into moving forward on his chosen path.

Then later, when Newt has reached the finish line, maybe he will become a proton ambassador, too (hint hint).

WHAT AMBASSADORS WANT FOR THEMSELVES

Al will do his best to help Newt, but Al's motivation is more complicated than meets the eye. What's in it for Al? Why did he choose to be a Proton Ambassador? The apparent answer is to help Newt, but Al is only human. He almost certainly has his own subconscious motivation that can influence his interaction with newbies.

We know why Newt called Al, and now we must explore the other side of the conversation. What motivates Al to speak with Newt, and what impression will he likely convey, consciously or not?

We ambassadors volunteered for the role because we remember what it was like to be a newbie and how much we appreciated the help we received from proton ambassadors. We are uniquely qualified to empathize with Newt, and now we want to pay it forward by helping to ease his suffering and provide a helpful, hopeful outlook. But we ambassadors are only human and as such, we often have our own possibly hidden or subconscious agenda.

While we certainly want to help Newt, is there more to the story?

Maybe so, but Newt is not wondering about our hidden agenda or underlying motivation for talking with him. He assumes our sole objective is to help him, and he is a thirsty sponge eagerly absorbing everything we dish out. He, and maybe also we ambassadors, are unaware that it is not so simple. This is unfortunate because understanding *our* more complex frame of mind should, but likely will not impact the way he interprets and digests what we tell him.

So, what do we tell him? On the surface, Al wants to address Newt's most obvious concerns head-on. His message as a proton ambassador will usually boil down to, "Proton works, and you are making a wise choice just like I did. So don't worry, it'll be fine." He sincerely believes this, it is probably true, and this is exactly what Newt is eager to hear.

Yet, like all of us, Al knows there is no treatment without risk, and proton is not perfect. But he does not readily point this out, nor does he intentionally omit it. After all, this tidbit of info is a downer and Al wants to be upbeat, so his comments naturally gravitate toward the happy and hopeful, not the risky and cautious. Furthermore, his statement is correct: everything probably *will* be fine. In most cases, the odds are heavily in Newt's favor. Why sully the promise of a likely positive outcome with a probably unnecessary caveat?

Al's message will be encouraging because intentionally or not, he will probably say what Newt wants to hear. After all, it is what Al wanted to hear when he was Newt. To help Newt feel less anxious, Al naturally tends to present a positive future full of promise, not a carefully measured scientific assessment of the statistical risks of various outcomes—precisely what Newt and ZapMe hope Al will do.

Even if Al had a less-than-perfect experience or outcome, his positive attitude is not dishonest. It is evidence of his survival instinct for self-preservation. For better or worse, every one of us must live with the irrevocable choices we make. There are no do-overs in the cancer treatment game. If things turned out well for Al, he is naturally a happy camper. But if his cancer is not brought under control or if the side effects are troublesome, what is he to do? Berate himself forever? Remain unhappy, bitter, and angry for life? Become a beacon of doom and gloom?

When the results are not perfect, most men, sometimes with great difficulty, will find a way to overcome any guilt or remorse they feel, as they must if they are to psychologically survive and lead a happy life. Creating a positive spin for a disappointing experience takes a lot of energy and effort, but once a man has done so it becomes integral to his thinking. Newt might hope for a brutally honest answer from such a man, but it is unfair and unrealistic to expect him to rekindle the negatives of his experience merely because he was asked. He has worked hard to bury the bad.

A prostate cancer survivor, even an ambassador, is not Wikipedia or WebMD. He is not merely an information source, but a player with skin in the game and feelings of his own. He cannot reasonably be expected to always provide unemotional, detached, objective, purely factual information. Ironically, answering Newt's questions also provides an opportunity for Al to reinforce his own well-honed positive view of *his* world. Sensitive, potentially embarrassing, or negative results might never arise in a newbie's conversation with him. Whether Al's experience was great or not so great, expecting complete objectivity and full disclosure from him may be wishful thinking.

Furthermore, let's face it: ambassador or not, we still maintain a modicum of modesty and a healthy dose of vanity. Unfortunately, the possible side effects of any prostate cancer treatment can feel embarrassing. We are not likely to say, "Hey, Newt! Everything is great except for my incontinence which has left me in diapers, but it's no big deal, you get used to it." This is not the image of us we want Newt to have, and we do not want this image of ourselves, despite its inevitability as we age with or without cancer.

Plus, Newt is not insensitive to Al's privacy, so he may hesitate to ask any potentially embarrassing, intrusive questions. When was the last time you asked any man whether he can still achieve an erection? It is an awkward question, and you can understand why Newt might not ask it.

With proton therapy, the results are overwhelmingly positive. Yet it is not without risk, and there are men who make the single-digit percentage risks of certain ill effects non-zero. My point here is not to highlight the likelihood or rarity of any particular outcome. It is to illustrate that with rare exception, proton ambassadors will have their own self-serving stories ranging from positive to ecstatic.

Ecstatic? Yes, proton ambassadors are sometimes extremely so. This is a bizarre and noteworthy phenomenon warranting further discussion.

POST-PROTON EUPHORIA

Now that you know why proton ambassadors generally tend to be so overly positive, I can highlight an unfortunate unintended consequence of being perhaps too upbeat in conversations with newbies. As you have seen, ambassadors often understandably make little to no mention of the risks, downplay any side effects they may have experienced, and amplify their positive results. Ironically, this overly positive message can backfire. When the cheerleading becomes too loud it begins to sound phony, or worse yet, desperate. When anything seems too good to be true, we rightfully begin to question its value.

Proton ambassadors—and I include myself here—are often guilty of this. Proton therapy has given most of us great results, and we want to tell the world. But I have often been told that we sound just too plain happy to be believable, especially during the first year or so after completing treatment. And it's true: As a group, we are indeed a bunch of happy if not giddy campers, and we don't try to hide it.

But this common and somewhat notorious post-proton euphoria does not go unnoticed. Once exposed to enough of it, Newt might start seeing our universal elation as extreme and insincere, as if we have all overdosed on some sort of proton happy-pill. He might wonder whether we are all on the payroll of our respective proton alma maters. *Surely proton therapy can't be that great*, Newt might justifiably think.

And he'd be right. Proton therapy is great, but not *that* great. Proton, along with every alternative cancer treatment, has risks including failure to control the cancer, future recurrence, and a standard list of side effects. We do not yet have a 100% perfect cure, no silver bullet for cancer killing. As incredible as proton is, especially as compared to other therapies, it is not yet perfect. It is merely amazing.

In explaining to Newt (or you) how I'm doing and whether I still believe proton therapy is the way to go, I am careful to avoid the ambassador trap of exhibiting excessive euphoria. I intentionally dial it down a notch, making certain he understands that although I am doing fine, I know proton men who have issues. The vast majority of the many proton men I've spoken with are doing very well, I will tell Newt. But not all of us, and it is important and only fair to at least mention this to Newt. Full disclosure, right?

Once diagnosed with prostate cancer, even when things go extremely well, we are saddled with new, unavoidable risks. They are inevitable, but manageable. We proton ambassadors will do a great service to a newbie by not only enthusiastically explaining the benefits of proton therapy, but also by helping him find a way to acknowledge and accept these inescapable uncertainties, and then navigate forward with realistic, sustainable optimism.

THE IMPACT OF ONE

Although a proton ambassador's post-proton euphoria can sometimes backfire, there may be an even greater chance of the opposite scenario. Newt and his fellow newbies are needy, and understandably so. When he repeatedly hears the glittering reports offered by us proton ambassadors, what if his thirst for hope and optimism causes Newt to take it too far? What if he inadvertently gives unwarranted significance to my stellar survivor status?

When Newt poses his "how are you doing" question to me, it is definitely not a light-hearted "how the heck are you, pal?" kind of question, and he is not looking for a quick "pretty darn good, thanks" answer. What Newt might really mean, the unstated question behind the question, is, "tell me how I'll be if I do what you did."

Let me state the obvious: How I am has next to nothing to do with how he will be. We know this and so does Newt, but we sometimes hear what we want to hear. Newt is desperately seeking encouragement, confidence, and reassurance that all will be well. He wants this so much that hearing a mere three words, "I'm doing fine," can become inflated into something entirely different in his vulnerable mind.

When those three magic words come from me, Newt's brain can easily translate them into a slippery slope of a logically flawed sequence more like, "Well, Ron's doing fine, he knows a lot of other guys who had proton, they're doing fine, the other proton men I've talked to are extremely enthusiastic, Ron sounds healthy and happy, they all sound amazingly upbeat, I want to be healthy and happy and upbeat, and yes indeed, I want to be one of those men so I should definitely have proton therapy because if it worked for them it'll work for me. Martha! I'm ready! Let's go!"

He is subconsciously using me as a surrogate for the man he may become after treatment, and he feels reassured by this very natural, but flawed transference. Of course, I do want to help Newt understand the benefits of proton therapy, as well as the risks. And I absolutely want to encourage him to seriously consider proton therapy to treat his prostate cancer. I also want him to know how well it worked for me. But quite frankly, I do not want to be the main reason he chooses proton, and I try to maneuver away from the euphoric "Martha, I'm ready" scenario.

Often, even this effort fails.

Ironically, by providing examples to remind Newt that despite my stellar results, proton is great but not perfect, my testimony can become even more impactful and believable. When Newt sees that I am fair-minded and forthright about not just the pros, but also the cons that indeed exist, he is often even more likely to feel good about proton therapy! My conscious effort to not convince him of anything backfires and achieves the opposite. It seems there is no way to avoid it.

I first experienced this bizarre phenomenon as a teenager when I had a thriving business giving guitar lessons. I recall one pleasant young student who had no talent, no technical ability, little interest, and was destined to suffer only frustration with his doomed pursuit. When I delicately explained this to his mother, suggesting that it might be more rewarding to explore other activities, her reaction astonished me. "Well, Ron," she said, "I appreciate your honesty, and because you are so honest, I would like him to continue guitar lessons with you. See you next week!" She completely missed the point, and I sometimes flash back to this example when attempting to be unbiased and realistic with newbies. The harder I try, the more accepting they seem to be.

Nevertheless, I do my best to remind Newt that no single example, including mine, can be used to predict what he should expect. His circumstances are different, and even if he is a perfect clone of me when I was diagnosed, his diagnosis follows at least a decade of medical advances. My options in 2010 were very good, but Newt's are better. Even proton therapy has improved.

Newt should be optimistic, but not merely because I did well. He can be justifiably hopeful because his diagnosis was today, not ten, twenty, or fifty years ago.

Newt's present may be challenging, but his future is bright.

As proton ambassadors, our main job is to do our best to convey this message of hope.

Epilogue

Epilogue sounds awfully melodramatic and maybe out of place in a book like this. But because I successfully fought the urge to have a prologue, I feel entitled to an epilogue to wrap things up in a tidy little bow.

First, I want to thank you for sticking with me to the finale, and I hope you had as much fun reading as I had telling my tale. As they say, that's my story and I'm sticking to it. The first part of my story is detailed in *PROTONS versus Prostate Cancer: EXPOSED*, written just after I completed proton therapy for prostate cancer in 2011. For those of you who read it, the book you are now holding is my follow-up, this time as a ten-year proton therapy veteran with enough time on his hands to write another book.

Much of what I have discussed here might equally apply to any kind of cancer. I suspect that these concepts could even be relevant in health challenges other than cancer, or to any unwelcome crisis thrown at us. But I'm only guessing. I cannot speak authoritatively about bladder cancer, heart disease, surviving an earthquake, or facing financial ruin. Maybe someday, but fortunately, not yet.

I have learned that unless you have walked the walk, you can only imagine the journey.

For me, it was and is prostate cancer, so that's what I write about in books and online. By sharing my experiences and insights as a proton therapy patient and prostate cancer survivor I hope to have given others on this path a guide rail to hold onto. It is a bumpy road, and we need all the help we can get.

I have come to terms with prostate cancer as a permanent part of my life, and this beast and I have a complex relationship. So far, I have the upper hand. As a survivor, I can speak with authority about my experience with it, and with proton therapy. I hope you have found my ten-year recap and insights useful, or at least occasionally amusing.

What's next for me? Who knows. I have toyed with the idea of writing a novel, or maybe a collection of slightly warped short stories for children. I also feel an increasing urge to refocus my life on music before the arthritis in my hands makes playing guitar a thing of the past, leaving me with only digital electronic music, not necessarily a bad option for an I.T. guy musician.

With other avenues of life to pursue and with limited time in this world, I know this could be my last book. That is, unless I reach my eighty-fifth birthday and write another one called *A Quarter-Century After Proton Therapy for Prostate Cancer.* But just to be safe, I felt I had better cram all the opinions I want to share into this one so my insights are not forever lost to the world, like my grandmother's recipe for porcupine balls, which I loved as a child and miss as an adult. If I could ask her just one more question, I would seek Nana's reason for taking the recipe with her to the grave.

Ah, sorry, my mind does wander (not a proton side effect, so don't worry). In any case, I do have a lot of opinions, many of which have changed in my post-cancer decade, and I don't want to take them to the grave. It is almost trite to say that cancer changes your life, but guess what: Cancer changes your life, and it's surprisingly often for the better. I believe I am a happier, wiser person than before cancer, and my cancer-curated views about life have matured. At last, my opinions might be worth sharing. At least some of them.

And here they are, recorded for you and for posterity. I hope you will take a moment to contact me and share your story and opinions so I will become even wiser, and my next book will be even better.

Finally, I would still like to have the recipe for Nana's porcupine balls. For me, they were right on target. Just like proton therapy.

Ron@AfterProton.com

Gratitude

I have a lot of good ideas. I also have many, many bad ones. In this book, you have seen a lot of the former and very few of the latter, and the reason is simple: Lucy.

After almost thirty years of marriage, my wonderful wife knows better than anyone exactly how my brain works. She can identify when it is performing well, and she relentlessly spots when it is not. In the privacy of our home, she sees plenty of both because here in my natural habitat, I am totally unfiltered.

Fortunately for you and luckily for me, Lucy has been willing to sift and screen my words before they travel beyond our humble abode. Most of what you have seen in my books, *The After Proton Blog*, and even some email and text messages have passed the rigorous Lucy Test. Admittedly, I sometimes ignore her advice and let my words sail away unfettered. Those passages or paragraphs in my writing that seem substandard, uninteresting, inappropriate, or possibly just plain dad-joke silly are almost certainly unfiltered, and I take full responsibility for allowing them through.

If my grammar, punctuation, and phrasing have improved, it is in part thanks to the education I received from Benjamin Dreyer in *Dreyer's English: An Utterly Correct Guide to Clarity and Style*. If you are a writer, aspire to be one, or happen to be a grammar geek, you will love this book. Dreyer has made an inherently dull and frustrating topic fun, mostly via candor and humor. Thank you, Ben. May I call you Ben?

And then there are my four fabulous daughters. Each is several notches smarter than I am, but I am smart enough to make use of their brilliance and talent when they let me. I invited them to proofread this book, as I did for my first one. Ten years ago Emily stepped up to the plate and skillfully edited my first endeavor. This time the editor's torch was passed to my oldest daughter Julie, an absolutely superb editor. Along with making many relatively minor corrections, she rescued me (and you) from a couple of major flaws, for which I am grateful. Julie's younger sister Jessica had her hand in both of my books, identifying inconsistencies, poor analogies, confusing passages, and unintended inferences. She helps me see not only the trees, but the forest. Last but not least is Caroline, my youngest, who contributed her talent as a graphic designer to create the perfect cover for this book. If the cover caught your eye, you can thank her.

Speaking of the cover, I must also thank my friend and professional photographer, Rick Smoak. You'll find the details of my experience with Rick in Appendix C ("The cover photos"), but he deserves a shoutout here as the guy who made this aging prostate cancer survivor look good not only on the cover, both front and back, but also in the "About the author" section. I have never looked as dignified as I do in Rick's photos, and if that weren't enough, he refused to bill me. However, I did buy him lunch. Once.

I also remain particularly grateful to three key doctors in my ten-year saga. First, Dr. Manny Venegas, my primary physician. He proactively checked my PSA, noted its rise in 2010, and sent me to Dr. Richard Morrow, a referral for which I will be forever grateful. Dr. Morrow is the fabled urologist fondly remembered by fans of Book#1 as "Dr. Pee," without whom you would not be reading this. He is the wonderful man who told me about proton therapy, urged me to investigate and consider it, and supported my decision to go for it. I sincerely thank you, Manny, for sending me to see Rick. With Venegas and Morrow I was batting two for two, lucky and lucky again.

I was lucky a third time to have found myself under the care of Dr. R. Charles Nichols, my oncologist at the University of Florida Health Proton Therapy Institute in Jacksonville. Along with being a highly skilled and experienced radiation oncologist, he is also an educator, taking the time to fully answer my many questions during my therapy and for years afterward. And I do tend to have a lot of questions. About everything. Sorry about that, Chip, but I hope you enjoyed our many chats even half as much as I did. I look forward to more. Yes, more. Sorry again.

Doctors Venegas, Morrow, and Nichols together kept me sane during the PSA roller coaster I described in this book, and I feel both lucky and grateful to have had their council. They each viewed my situation through their own unique lens, and the combined result was exactly what I needed. At each annual wellness checkup Dr. Venegas reassuringly showed little if any concern about my cancer because from his primary-physician point of view, a PSA of 3 was normal enough. Dr. Nichols, with a sharp eye on my prostate and a furrowed brow at PSA 3, began prudently painting possible avenues to pursue if things went south. Dr. Morrow, ever the realist, provided a calming country-doctorish perspective, bridging the gap between laissez-faire and terror-driven approaches, guiding me forward at the right pace with a measured, unpanicked level of concern. With the help of these three wise men, I finally disembarked from the roller coaster in one piece physically and mentally.

If I learned a lot from this elite triumvirate of physicians, I have been equally educated throughout the years by my many proton brothers. We have had lengthy conversations from which I gained vicarious experience beyond my own, and achieved correspondingly greater wisdom, hopefully reflected in this book. I also began new friendships strengthened by the bond we share as fellow travelers on a road we never imagined navigating. Many thanks to you, my proton brothers. We were, are, and will continue to be in this together.

Finally, although it was not the topic of this book, I simply must include my appreciation for those who made it possible for me to have proton therapy in 2011. First on that list are the geniuses at IBA (Ion Beam Applications). They conceived, manufactured, sold, delivered, and maintained the equipment that fired an undisclosed number of protons precisely into the target—my prostate. Most of their work is done behind the scenes without much direct patient contact, which strikes me as sad because without them, there would have been no protons for me. Whether the proton equipment that zapped you boasted IBA's logo or that of one of their competitors, I know we can all clap our hands loudly to thank these technical wizards for the magic machines that made our cancer disappear. Go ahead. Clap now.

Last in line, but foremost in mind, are all the people at my proton alma mater, the University of Florida Health Proton Therapy Institute in Jacksonville. The warm welcomers in the Intake Department, the many compassionate doctors, nurses, and radiation therapists, the smiling receptionists, the thankless volunteers, and the conscientious administrative staff, all watching out for little old me before, during, and after proton therapy—thank you for making this decade not only successful, but packed full of amazing memories.

If you were treated in my era, 2010 or before, there is a good chance you were also treated at UF Proton because way back then, there were only a handful of proton facilities in the country. Today there are dozens of excellent centers, so odds are you were or will be treated somewhere closer to your home. And just as I have an obvious affinity and appreciation for my proton alma mater, I expect you will feel the same about yours. They are our heroes. Kudos to them all.

As proton therapy centers have proliferated, they have generally maintained a highly patient-centric approach to cancer treatment. They have learned from each other, modeled their methodology after the most successful centers, and come together annually when the National Association of Proton Therapy holds a conference to discuss the past, present, and future of proton therapy. While we will each have a special fondness for our own proton alma mater, we can all appreciate how our greater community has grown from the early days (1990) of a lone proton center in Loma Linda, California.

May the growth continue!

Finally, I thank *you* for sticking with me to the end of my ten-year brain dump. I hope you found something of value here. The only reason I wrote this book was so you could read it, so thanks for making it worth the effort. Now send me an email and make my day!

Maybe I'll see you again in my book#3, *A Quarter-Century After Proton Therapy for Prostate Cancer*. I'm a slow writer, so I suppose I should start writing it now.

APPENDIX A:
My PSA Chart

I now present to you my glorious PSA chart, divided into two halves, before and after proton, for easier reading. I offer this data for your amusement only. Please do not make any medical inferences from it that might influence the decisions you are facing. This is my chart. Yours will be different.

Also, in full disclosure, my PSA popped to 9.3 on the last day of my proton therapy. They test within a day of graduation for completeness, but the reading on that day doesn't mean much. A quick post-therapy spike is common and virtually without significance. After all, at that moment my prostate was highly agitated after being relentlessly zapped 39 times! It is easy to understand why there might be a resulting brief spike, sort of the prostate's way of shouting, "Yikes!"

I omitted the yikes-spike from these charts because it would flatten the rest of the line, making it needlessly difficult for you to see the pattern of ups and downs I experienced, the roller coaster I described earlier in detail. Just know that there was an insignificant spike between the two charts.

First, for my fellow numbers-nerds, is the raw data. Then the charts.

Enjoy.

PSA BEFORE PROTON THERAPY		
Date	PSA	Up/Down from prior
1999-04	1.6	first PSA test
2004-12	3.0	↑
2007-03	3.8	↑
2008-03	3.7	↓
2008-09	4.5	↑
2008-11	4.4	↓
2009-01	4.2	↓
2009-03	4.2	(same)
2009-09	4.8	↑
2010-03	5.1	↑
2010-04	5.1	(same)
2010-09	5.9	↑
2010-12	5.8	↓

PSA AFTER PROTON THERAPY		
Date	PSA	Up/Down from prior
2011-06	2.6	↓
2011-09	2.1	↓
2011-12	1.3	↓
2012-03	1.2	↓
2012-06	1.7	↑
2012-09	1.2	↓
2013-03	1.4	↑
2013-09	2.3	↑
2014-03	1.3	↓
2014-09	1.8	↑
2014-10	1.4	↓
2015-03	2.3	↑
2015-10	2.1	↓
2016-02	3.0	↑
2016-06	1.3	↓
2016-12	1.2	↓
2017-06	1.4	↑
2018-02	1.0	↓
2018-08	0.8	↓
2019-03	0.9	↑
2019-09	0.8	↓
2020-03	0.9	↑
2020-09	0.8	↓
2021-03	0.8	(same)
2021-09	0.8	(same)

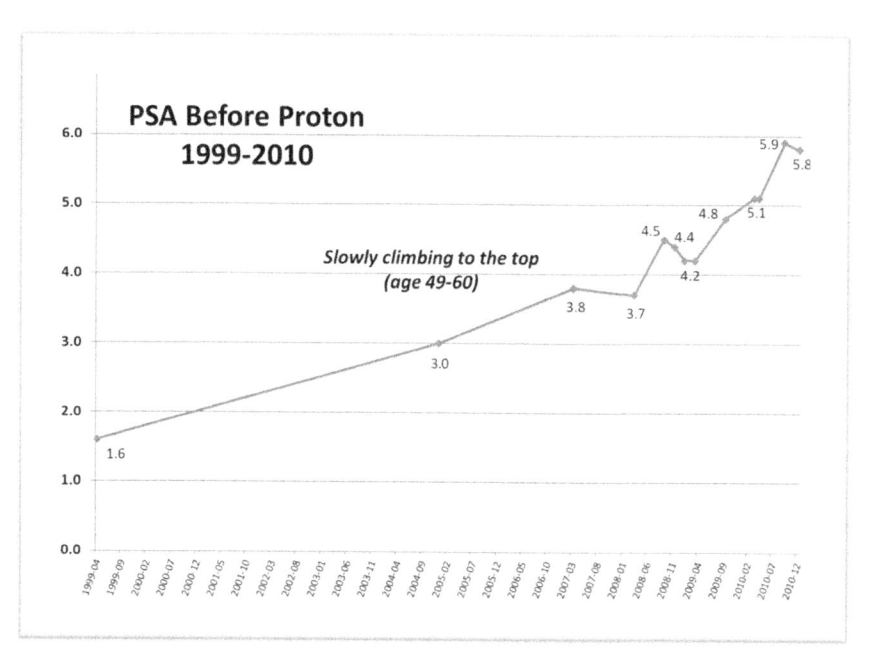

PSA Before Proton 1999-2010

Slowly climbing to the top (age 49-60)

Date	PSA
1999-04	1.6
2004-09	3.0
2007-03	3.8
2008-01	3.7
2008-06	4.5
2008-11	4.4
2009-04	4.2
2009-09	4.8
2010-02	5.1
2010-07	5.9
2010-12	5.8

PSA After Proton 2011-Present

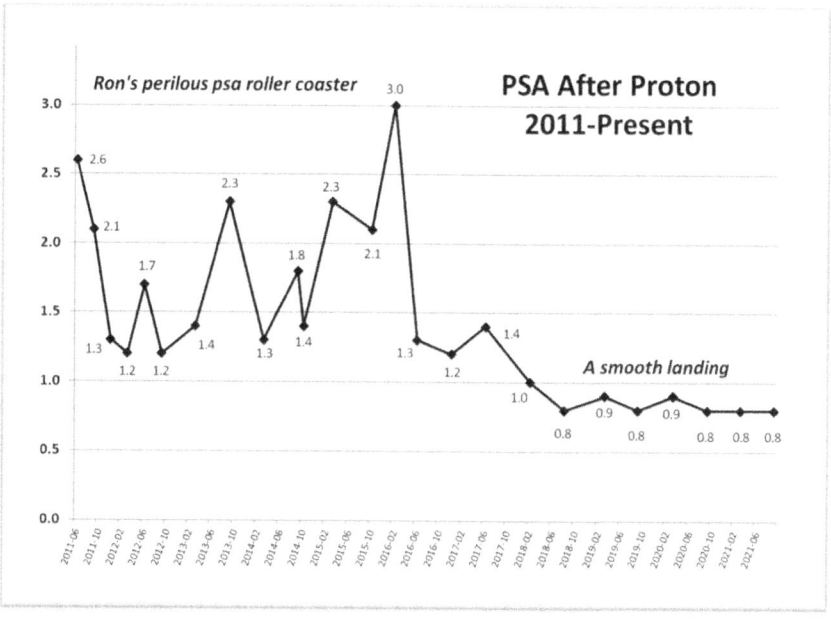

Ron's perilous psa roller coaster

A smooth landing

Date	PSA
2011-06	2.6
2011-10	2.1
2012-02	1.3
2012-06	1.7
2012-10	1.2
2013-06	1.2
2013-10	1.4
2014-02	2.3
2014-06	1.3
2014-10	1.4
2015-02	1.8
2015-06	2.3
2015-10	2.1
2016-02	3.0
2016-06	1.3
2016-10	1.2
2017-02	1.4
2017-06	1.4
2017-10	1.0
2018-02	0.8
2018-06	0.9
2018-10	0.8
2019-02	0.9
2019-06	0.8
2020-02	0.8
2020-06	0.8
2020-10	0.8
2021-02	0.8
2021-06	0.8

APPENDIX B:
My 11-Year Update

Looking at the timeline for the evolution of this book, I have validated my credentials as a super-slow writer. I began writing *10 Years After* when it was really only 9 years, and lo and behold, it is now more than 11. Taking the average, I suppose 10 is still a reasonable book title.

But in the time it took me to complete all the other chapters, the world and my life have undergone some notable changes that deserve mention. Rather than revise what I have already written to reflect those changes, I will leave well enough alone. Instead, I will summarize them all here in a separate chapter devoted to year 11.

Then I will do my best to publish this before any other big changes occur. As I said, I am a slow writer.

MY HEALTH

I have reread the second chapter, "My 10-Year Health Checkup," and now, after another year or so, everything thankfully still applies, along with a few additions of minor importance, depending on your point of view.

I have less hair on my head, but with concentrated effort and surgical precision I can still manage to make it look … okay. The color has changed, and I'm hoping we can agree to say it's more dignified looking now. Sure, why not. Let's say *that*. In any case, Lucy assures me that nobody cares about my hair. Her words. So be it.

My vision is still pretty good, although my eye doctor says cataracts are developing. I have a new pair of glasses for the first time in a long time. Lucy says the new frames make me look ten years younger, which seems a little like pointing out that someone has lost weight. I'm not totally sure how to interpret her remark, but regardless, I wear the glasses even when I don't need them. Wouldn't you?

I am learning about arthritis, particularly in the fingers of my right hand. It is most noticeable in the morning and not much of an issue during the day, but probably going to get worse before it gets better, if it ever does. And just to make sure my right hand didn't get all the attention, I cut the index finger of my left hand with a box blade while cutting a box. Not very creative, I know. The cut required three stitches and injured or possibly cut the radial nerve. My finger is still recovering but will not likely reach 100% of its old self. Well, that's par for the course: few parts of my body resemble their old selves anymore. Thankfully, the nerve damage does not seem to impair my ability to play guitar, although some things feel a little strange and will take some getting used to. And I will get used to it. I have acclimated to worse things than a finicky finger, as I have already enumerated in detail.

Finally, I am now seventy-two years old, into year twelve post-proton. But the book title will remain unchanged because it somehow sounds better than *11 Years After*.

THE COVID-19 PANDEMIC

I hope the Covid-19 pandemic will have become just a bad memory by the time you read this, but it was in full swing, toilet paper shortages and all, while writing this book. Like many others, I have a growing list of Pandemic Postponements, some voluntary and others mandatory.

My 9-year checkup in Jacksonville never happened. It was scheduled for the last week in March 2020, just a couple of weeks after pandemic lockdowns began. I expected the world to have returned to normal before my big 10-year milestone, and so did UF Proton. But no, the pandemic was still raging and in 2021 I missed yet another southbound celebration. For number ten I was scheduled to see my oncologist, make two presentations to the radiation therapists, speak at the prostate cancer clinic, and have dinner with some good friends on the UF Proton staff. All sadly canceled. (Now that I say this, maybe Lucy is right again. Maybe I am pro-proton. Hmmm.) I had no Jacksonville visit in 2022, either. Surely by March 2023?

I have not yet returned to Jacksonville because Covid-19 remains a threat, and as a good South Carolinian, I want to neither import nor export it state-to-state. Thankfully, with a PSA of 0.8 I have no urgent reason to see my oncologist, or even my local urologist. I continue to see my local primary physician for checkups and to monitor my vital signs and blood levels, so I am confident of being okay. I did see my gastro guy for a Covid-delayed colonoscopy, which thankfully also turned out fine, or at least as fine as a colonoscopy can be.

I remain a retired, mostly stay-at-home man, and while the pandemic caused relatively minor inconvenience for me, it dramatically changed the modus operandi for patients diagnosed or treated during this period. Some postponed a biopsy, and many delayed treatment just to avoid the risks of travel, crowds, and medical facilities. Thankfully, with close monitoring, the slow-growing nature of prostate cancer allows some delay of treatment without much additional risk, which is fortunate for those faced with such difficult choices beyond the normal ones.

For those who did obtain treatment during the pandemic, the experience was markedly different than mine, as I fully described it in Book#1. The necessary keep-your-distance, lockdown paradigm made it more difficult, though not impossible, to achieve the same special bond between proton brothers, and the social support I enjoyed in 2011 was harder to come by. I hope things will improve soon so future patients can have their version of the amazing experience that inspired my first book. In the meantime, patients during the pandemic will still have the medical benefits of proton but will have to try a little harder for the social benefits.

And it will be worth it.

PROTON THERAPY

I am going to deviate from my plan for this book and delve into some semi-technical topics related to proton therapy in 2022. It's exciting, and I find that I simply cannot resist using a few pages for a brief mention of the highlights of how proton therapy has evolved not only since I began this Book#2, but since I was treated in

2011. After all, this *is* the "update" chapter in a book about me, and I had proton therapy, so why not include at least a brief update on that?

But I will resist going down the deep rabbit hole of detailed explanations. I encourage you to dig further on your own to whatever degree you are interested. You can use this chapter as a starting point for further research to keep you busy on a rainy day.

Of course, by the time you read this, my proton therapy update information will likely have evolved even further. Nevertheless, I have decided to include it as a marker-in-time to describe the state of proton at the time of publication, and to provide proof that proton technology is indeed marching onward.

Hypofractionation vs. radiation vacations

A decade ago, and to some extent even now, the standard of treatment for proton radiation for prostate cancer was to deliver 78 gray (a unit of measurement for radiation) in 39 sessions, which is exactly what I received. Those were the good old days, when prostate cancer proton patients were awarded with a two-month hiatus from their daily grind. For most, those eight weeks, often away from home, involved a little bit of radiation, a lot of golf, and priceless camaraderie with fellow patients. This wonderfully unique and special experience came to be affectionately known as their "radiation vacation." Clever. Wish I had coined the phrase.

Since then, clinical trials have shown that various degrees of hypofractionation (i.e., fewer, larger doses) are equally, or possibly even more safe and effective. Nowadays it is not uncommon to receive only 28 slightly higher-dose zaps. A 20-zap protocol is also being tested, and some clinics offer proton radiation in a 5-dose SBRT (stereotactic body radiotherapy) protocol. Almost unbelievably, it even looks like what is now called "flash" therapy holds the promise of treating prostate cancer with just one or two outpatient proton blasts.

Radiation vacations may soon become a thing of the past.

Scatter beam vs. pencil beam

Proton therapy for prostate cancer has evolved in other ways. For the first quarter century of its use in the United States, protons were typically delivered using one of several variations of a technique called "scatter beam." To treat my prostate in 2011, the original thin beam of protons first passed through a brass modulator to make it wider, followed by an acrylic range compensator to vary the beam's depth. Together, these two devices shaped the beam to fit my three-dimensional prostate. Because the compensator and modulator are custom-made to fit the precise size and shape of each patient's prostate, they cannot be reused. However, the brass is melted and recycled, and the acrylic prostate-shaped bowl is offered to the patient as a parting gift, presumably put to good use as a fancy dish for M&Ms or guacamole dip. No joke, and yes, some people find this to be a little creepy.

Another proton technology called "pencil beam scanning," or PBS, is coming into widespread use. With this method there is no need for a modulator or compensator, so the time, cost, and logistics associated with those devices are eliminated. With PBS, the thin beam is steered with magnets and is used like a pencil, coloring in the prostate with a back-and-forth motion at varying depths until the entire target is precisely covered. While both scatter beam and PBS are still used effectively for prostate cancer, there are some cancers for which pencil beam scanning has significant advantages. Brain tumors, particularly in children, are at the top of this list that includes head, neck, eyes, throat, spine, and other cancers.

My descriptions of scatter beam and pencil beam scanning are oversimplifications of complex technology, but you should now have a general idea of how they work. This understanding should also serve to illustrate that with any treatment modality including proton therapy, there is no *one-size-fits-all* approach. There are options within options. If you are on the road to proton now, be sure to check into the details of hypofractionation, scatter beam, pencil beam, and any new variations introduced after this book was published.

Also consider balloons versus SpaceOAR.

Balloons and SpaceOAR™

Is proton therapy for prostate cancer so festive that we celebrate with balloons? And is a SpaceOAR some kind of high-tech paddle? Well, no and no. As my balloon brethren know, we are talking about rectal balloons, not party decorations. And as the new breed of gel-guys know, the SpaceOAR Hydrogel system is a newer alternative that does much the same job as balloons, with some advantages. But are balloons now obsolete? Is the infamous rectal balloon destined to gradually fade away along with radiation vacations? Again, no and no.

Rectal balloons and the SpaceOAR System both address two important concerns during radiotherapy for prostate cancer: stabilizing the prostate and protecting the rectum. Neither balloons nor SpaceOAR are perfect solutions, but they provide equally clever yet very different ways to effectively tackle these issues. With just a few keys and clicks on your computer, you can easily find the technical details of how they work. What you will not find elsewhere is the extraordinarily concise, bottom line, one-paragraph description and comparison of balloons and SpaceOAR, available only here:

A specialized balloon can be inserted into the rectum and plumped up with saline, thereby pushing the rectum against the prostate to stabilize it while keeping most of the rectum out of the field of radiation. Alternatively, the SpaceOAR Hydrogel can be injected via the perineum into the fatty corridor between the rectal wall and prostate, creating a protective safe zone between the two, and significantly reducing or eliminating radiation exposure to the rectum while also providing some stabilization of the prostate. A balloon is used before each therapy session and then discarded; the hydrogel is injected in a one-time procedure a few days before therapy begins and is later absorbed into the body within a few months. The balloon does a better job stabilizing the prostate, while the gel is superior at protecting the rectum.

Of course, balloons are undeniably more festive and fun. As a newbie, you are probably trying to imagine the balloon experience, but don't bother, it's nearly impossible. If you really want to know, all the intimate details are in Book#1 where I devoted an entire chapter to it, and there's no need to repeat it here. Suffice it to say it is a weirdly disturbing unique sensation, but not painful, and after a few dozen times it becomes old hat.

What does the gel feel like? I cannot speak about this from personal experience. I considered having the injection as research for this book, but insurance would not cover it as an author expense. Instead, I spoke with some gel guys. Most report minimal sensation during the injection, typically with only a local anesthetic. Only a few mentioned occasional discomfort bordering on pain during or after the brief procedure. Some men experience a "full" sensation while the gel is in place. More frequent or urgent urination could also result from the pressure the gel applies against the prostate, which in turn presses on the bladder, our notorious urine reservoir. For the most part, life with the gel is normal enough, and in a casual meeting you cannot distinguish a new era gel-guy from a balloon-boy like me.

For now, SpaceOAR rules the roost and has largely supplanted the old reliable rectal balloons. This is generally regarded as good news not only by newbies, but also by our beloved radiation therapists who I am certain would enthusiastically thank the FDA for approving SpaceOAR for prostate cancer in 2015. On that day, RTs throughout the U.S.A. could be heard loudly shouting with glee as they rejoiced and welcomed this innovation. Before then, the RT who drew the short straw had the questionable privilege of gently sliding a rectal balloon into our derriere before each zap. Well, those days are nearly gone.

Nearly, but not totally. Some men will not qualify for SpaceOAR. An enlarged prostate, insufficient space between the prostate and rectum, or pre-existing urinary issues are some of the potential disqualifiers. For them, it is back to the tried-and-true balloons. Also, if the gel is already in use and the prostate nevertheless moves around more than SpaceOAR can handle, balloons might be called upon to save the day. That's right, some lucky guys will get both SpaceOAR and balloons.

The use of SpaceOAR is sOARing, but the balloon has not gone bust, so you RTs should keep those straws handy, just in case.

More proton facilities

Although not quite yet matching the level of Starbucks, the number of proton centers is growing in the US and the world. In 2010 there was just a handful in the US, and now there are dozens. I see articles almost every day about the next one proposed, under construction, or about to open. There are some good reasons for this increased interest in providing proton beam therapy.

First and foremost, proton therapy works, and the word is out. When cancer calls, people often want proton if they are lucky enough to know about it. I know I am repeating myself when I tell you that as compared with conventional x-ray/photon radiation, proton therapy delivers less radiation to healthy tissue, thus reducing the risks of side effects or secondary cancers down the road. This makes it worth considering for any cancer, but for some cancers the precision of proton therapy makes it the only viable option.

Bottom line: patients want it.

As much as it would be nice to have a handy proton center on every corner, there have been two major obstacles to building one: high cost and large footprint. The size of early facilities was often compared to a football field, and such real estate is hard to come by, especially in a convenient location near the population to be served. Plus, the investment was significant, carrying a hefty price tag in the hundreds of millions. Even if a medical facility wanted to add proton capability, where would they put it? And how would they pay for it?

The good news is that those impediments have been reduced. While it is sometimes still beneficial to build large facilities with several treatment rooms, there is a new option. Today, a single-room compact proton facility, cyclotron and all, can be constructed with a much smaller footprint and significantly lower price tag. This might even fit entirely within an existing cancer center, with minimal or no additional land required.

Many cancer treatment centers are taking advantage of this development, and finding a proton center close to home is more of a possibility than ever before. In 2011 I felt very lucky to have a reputable proton facility within a five-hour drive of my home, and today many more patients can say the same.

I realize this ten-year update of proton therapy—hypofractionation, scatter beam, pencil beam, balloons, SpaceOAR, increased access—has been more technical, and contrary to the stated objective of this book. But once I got here, it felt odd not to at least pay homage to those developments. I hope you will regard it as added value, not worthless wandering.

But now it's back to the personal point of the book, and the 11-year update of my life after proton. Having paid adequate attention to proton therapy advances, I now wish to pay homage to a dear friend.

LESSONS LEARNED FROM A DOG

Baxter, the only dog I have had in my adult life, died on February 13, 2021. He was very much alive when I began this book, and I have already mentioned him more than once. I can fill a few pages with my memories of him, but I will never be able to fill the empty place in my heart that he once occupied. I miss Baxter every day, and he deserves some pages here for several reasons.

I do realize that you might regard this chapter as self-indulgent, and if so, that's fine with me. You would be perfectly justified in feeling that devoting any number of pages in a book about cancer to my dog is inappropriate and irrelevant. Well, if that happens to be how you feel, I will respectfully disagree. My decade of life after proton therapy for prostate cancer would have been quite different without Baxter.

Lucy and I inherited this amazing mutt from my mother-in-law when she died just a few months after I completed proton therapy in 2011. Baxter was destined to be my daily companion for the ten years after proton, the decade this book is about. And he taught me a lot, not only about how strong and meaningful the bond between a person and a dog can be, but also about life. I attribute some of my personal growth during this time to my relationship with this remarkable creature.

I was lucky to have Baxter at my side, as a constant companion during the ten years post-proton. His portrait by painter Heather LaHaise, a wonderful birthday gift from Lucy in 2017, hangs on my office wall directly behind my computer monitor. Seeing his image elicits fond memories and a smile along with a heavy heart and a few tears, even now.

I shared my thoughts and feelings about Baxter online twice. The first article, "Two Old Dogs After Proton Therapy," was written in 2019, just before Baxter had two major back-to-back seizures that almost killed him. I wrote the second article, "Just a Dog—My Apology," a few days after his death. It is somewhat of a eulogy for Baxter and a catharsis for me.

Rather than paraphrasing either article, I will share both here as they were published online, photos and all. By reading them, I hope you will benefit a bit from Baxter's life through my words.

Baxter, you were the best.

Two Old Dogs After Proton Therapy
August 9, 2019

My beloved mother-in-law died just three months after I completed proton therapy for prostate cancer at the University of Florida Health Proton Therapy Institute in Jacksonville. On that day we inherited and adopted Baxter, the perky little 27-pound mutt who kept her company in her final years. Baxter and I have been best pals ever since, and he has taught me a lot about life—lessons that are particularly valuable in my post-proton, post-cancer existence.

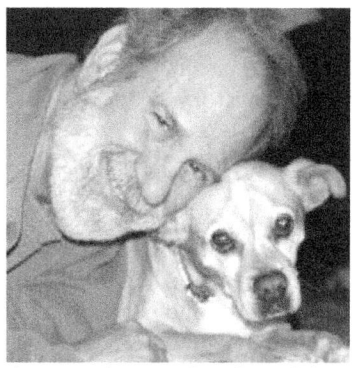

Baxter was then (2010) about six years old and I was sixty, ten times his age in absolute years, but only about fifty percent older using the seven-dog-years-per-human-year formula. Today (2019) I am sixty-nine and Baxter just turned fifteen. That makes me 4.6 times his age in absolute years, but using dog years he is now older than me by about twenty percent.

So who is older? And does it really matter? Any way you look at it, we're just a couple of old dogs muddling through life.

Our checkups

Yesterday he had a "senior" medical checkup at the one place on earth into which he must be carried. He now perceives those telltale double-glass doors as the portal to a canine torture chamber. He understandably resists, and I can no longer even push him in. Thankfully, he's still under thirty pounds and I can carry him. Of course, Baxter has never been hurt at the vet, but it is nevertheless no fun and causes him anxiety.

When it's over I reward him with his favorite treat, and he's happy again.

I can relate to how he feels. My anxiety level spikes every time I have a blood draw, which is literally a hit-and-miss proposition. I may soon require someone to carry me into the lab tech's office. Once they eventually get what they need, my focus shifts to concern about what the results might mean for me—a second level of anxiety Baxter is spared. Even almost nine years post-proton, PSA anxiety still lingers.

Although I do reward myself with a treat (typically a Hardee's cinnamon raisin biscuit), I'm not totally happy again until I know my lab results are satisfactory.

Our health status

How's Baxter doing? He's doing very well "for an old dog." There's some arthritis in his left hind leg, he's lost most of his hearing, his vision is a tad cloudy, and his alkaline phosphate level is too high for a healthy gall bladder.

But only his veterinarian knows any of this, and only she knows that his gall bladder has lost some structural integrity. The only outwardly visible evidence of Baxter's age is his grayer, whiter hair, a couple extra pounds, and a flappy loose-fitting jowl under his chin.

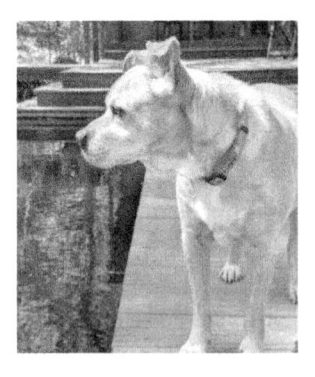

Overall, he appears to be a pretty darn healthy dog.

How am I doing? Very well "for a man my age." I have some arthritis in my shoulders, I've lost some hearing in the upper frequencies, I have floaters in both eyes, a whistle in my left ear, and restricted air flow in my right nostril. Of course, you can see none of this.

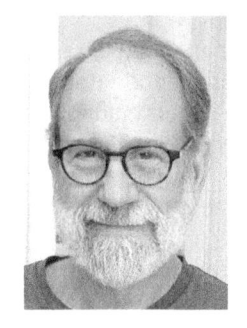

Nor can you see that my prostate is a flattened, toughened, barely functional mass of proton-radiated (cancer-free) tissue—something only my oncologist has seen (or more accurately, felt). The only outward evidence of my age is a salt-and-pepper beard that was black for many decades, grayer and sparser hair on my head under my hat, and an excess amount of me in my midsection.

Overall, I appear to be a pretty darn healthy guy.

Our clocks

Baxter and I have a lot in common, but we differ completely when it comes to our sense of time. He lives in the present and is totally focused on the moment at hand. He is aware of no past, nor a future. He does this naturally—didn't even need to attend a mindfulness class for senior canines. Saved me a lot of money.

I do my best to emulate him, but I cannot devote all my time to "being present." The past lingers forever, and the future requires planning. I am working to improve my ability to ignore the bygones and yet-to-comes of my life while fully enjoying the moment, but it still takes effort. How nice it would be to have a Baxter-Button that would switch my focus at will.

Baxter's recent medical checkup provides a perfect illustration of our different perception of time. His appointment was close to noon and his labs required fasting. I said to my wife Lucy, "This is horrible. Baxter is going to hate me. He won't understand why I'm depriving him of his breakfast and morning treats. He'll think he did something wrong, that he disappointed me and lost my love. He'll never forgive me for rejecting him!" To be sure, Baxter was a little hungry and confused for a few hours, but it was torture for me.

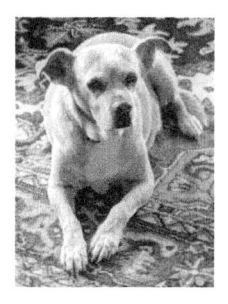

Lucy accurately assured me that once I fed Baxter we'd be pals again, and he'd never even be able to recall the brief deprivation. There would be no "remember the time you starved me all morning" recrimination, no lingering lack of trust or love. There'd be no forgiveness because there'd be nothing to forgive. It would be as if it had never happened. No wallowing in the past, no worrying whether it will happen again. It's so easy for him.

Our walks in the woods

Nearly every morning Baxter and I take a leisurely walk in the woods. It's not as lengthy as in younger days, nor as vigorous, but it's every bit as wonderful and important to us both. Without a leash, Baxter leads the way through the trees, pridefully prancing as the lead dog, exuding joyfulness with every step. I focus on him and feel fortunate to have yet another day to share the moment, enjoying his company and appreciating the beauty that surrounds us. It is a much-needed morning meditation that impacts the remainder of my day.

As Baxter's student, I observe that he stops to sniff every interesting scent he encounters, never lamenting his inability to hear what he so adeptly detects with his nose. He stops frequently, sticking his snout into a pile of leaves or a patch of grass, inhaling the cacophony of aromas for many minutes, unconcerned about delaying our progress. He has taught me to patiently wait and vicariously appreciate his thorough olfactory analysis. Only when he's satisfied that his inspection is complete does he forge ahead. He now huffs and puffs while slowly traversing the inclines of our path, never seeming to suffer or care about his diminished stamina or arthritic legs.

For him, this is how it is, and it's pretty darn good.

I take my cue from him. The sounds of the birds, the wind, the rustling trees, and the crunching beneath my boots create a symphony of calm. I'm happy to hear these sounds, even without the upper frequencies I'm now missing, and even with the persistent whistle in my head. To a far lesser degree than Baxter, I can also enjoy the surrounding scents—even without much help from my restricted right nostril. And the visual beauty is ever-changing and breathtaking, forcing the floaters that faintly speckle my vision into the background.

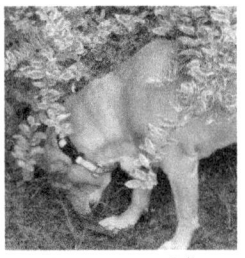

For me, this is how it is, and it's pretty great.

With the help of Baxter, at least on our walks I live in the present. I do my best to retain and apply that ability for the rest of the day. After all, the present is all I am assured of having. It's life, and I don't want to miss it.

Old dogs

We are indeed a couple of old dogs—at least old enough to have had things happen that I wish had not. Tinnitus, lost frequencies, floaters, and a touch of cancer—I didn't want any of those, but I've learned to live with them. They were all surprises that should not have surprised me because clearly, this is how life works. Stuff happens. It's not "if," it's "what and when."

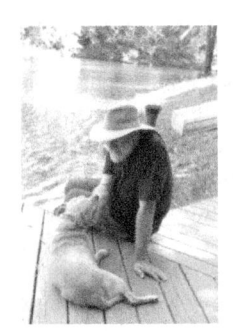

I know and accept that more stuff will happen to both me and Baxter, guaranteed. Some good, some ... meh. Eventually something will end it all, hopefully quickly and painlessly. Either of us could be hit by a bus—end of story. Baxter's gall bladder could stop doing its job. I could encounter a new or returning cancer or an entirely different and possibly worse illness, making my remaining life more of a challenge. It will assuredly be something. I just don't know what or when.

Does it really matter? Absolutely, but I'll follow Baxter's carefree lead as much as I can. I'll endeavor to notice and appreciate the good things in each moment to whatever degree I can. It's the only approach that makes sense.

Especially for an old dog.

Just a Dog—
My Apology
February 26, 2021

This one is not about prostate cancer or prostate therapy. This is my confession and apology to dog people everywhere. I'll include cat people, too, assuming their experience may be similar, but I'll restrict my references to dogs.

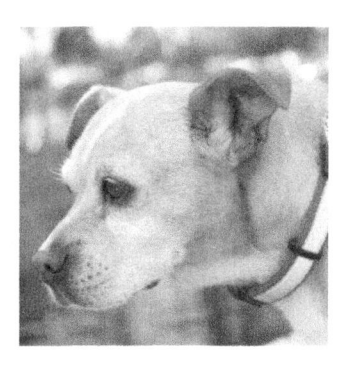

I have often heard dog owners refer to their pets as "my kids" or "my little girl" or "my boy" and the like, and it has always struck me as slightly strange if not totally bizarre. After all, I told myself, they are referring to dogs, not small humans. It seemed to me that using such terminology undeservedly bestowed near-human status to a mere animal. Furthermore, it made the owner seem a little silly. After all, a dog is just a dog.

And how much is a dog worth, anyway? How many dollars is it reasonable to relinquish for what sometimes appeared to me to be a dog's excessive creature comforts? Exotic beds, clothes, travel gear, cuisine, and such. And if injured or seriously sick, why would people spend thousands of dollars to keep their dog ticking along for a few more months or years? No animal should be mistreated, but why not just get another dog?

I mean, really. It's just a dog, right?

If you are already outraged at the views expressed above, well, so am I. I am horrified that they were mine. I believe and hope I have largely kept such judgmental stupidity to myself but fear I may have occasionally made comments aloud. If I have ever directed such thoughts or words toward you, I now wish to apologize publicly and profusely.

Sadly, now I get it.

It has been ten days since my 16½-year-old dog Baxter took his last breath, and only now am I able to talk about it. I know many of you have experienced the loss of a beloved pet, and nothing I say here will be news to you. That's okay because I'm writing this largely for me, for Baxter, for anyone who knew him, and for all who are willing to hear his story.

An unexpected gift

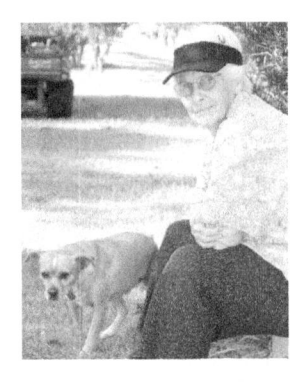

In 2008 my widowed mother-in-law Laura was living about a mile from my home. Around that time my wife's cousin Betty decided Laura needed a dog. Betty knew a family with a dozen dogs, and Baxter was low man on the totem pole. So they gave Baxter to Betty, and Betty unceremoniously plunked him down on Laura's lawn saying, "You need a dog. Here you go. See ya later." Despite her initial objections, Baxter became Laura's dog, and they soon learned to appreciate each other quite well.

With our frequent visits there, Lucy and I became fond of Baxter, and when my mother-in-law died in 2011 (just three months after I completed proton therapy), we happily inherited him. However, Lucy and I had already discussed having a dog and agreed it wouldn't work with our lifestyle. Plus, neither of us had ever had a dog in our adult lives. So Baxter's arrival was met with both of us asking, "What do we do now?"

Well of course, we figured it out. Baxter had always been blissfully happy as strictly an outside dog—very common in rural areas—which made our role relatively simple. We made a warm place for him in the garage, put a well-outfitted doghouse on the porch, placed bowls of water in several convenient locations, and fed him the same food he was accustomed to in the same bowl he had always used. And with each passing day, we loved him a little more.

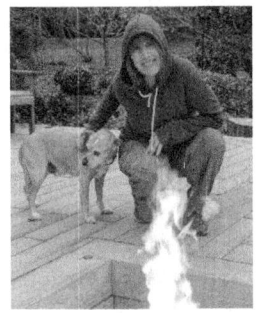

In our first years with Baxter Lucy did the lion's share of caring for her mom's dog, now ours, including all the fun stuff as well as the not-so-fun. But when I retired in 2015 and Lucy continued to be gainfully employed, it logically fell to me to pick up the ball, and after about five years of observing her, I fell into the role quickly enough.

And I loved it. Baxter made it so easy. I do not exaggerate by saying he never did anything wrong, never needed our training or reprimand, and somehow always knew what to do and what not to do. He was a perfect and constant companion for me during retirement. We religiously took a morning walk in the woods or around the pond, or pretty much wherever he wanted to lead me. It was the high point of his day, and always started me off on the right foot, like a morning meditation.

He was eager to ride shotgun when I drove the quarter mile to take out the trash, and I extended the ride just so he could enjoy the wind on his face a little longer. I'm not sure which of us enjoyed it more.

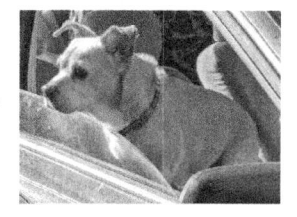

Outside-in

I would never have expected Baxter's gradual transformation from being a totally outside dog to a completely inside one. We first brought him into the house to temporarily monitor his recovery after an injury requiring the infamous "cone of shame." He used the opportunity to demonstrate that he could be a perfect inside dog, too, and we all kind of liked it.

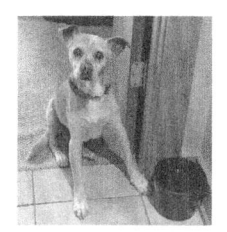

With his foot in the door, he still remained mostly an outside dog, coming in for occasional variety whenever he wished through the new doggie door we provided. As he grew older, Baxter seemed to increasingly appreciate the creature comforts of the inner sanctum. He gradually became mostly an inside dog, which we all enjoyed immensely.

After a while, on a whim I put him on my lap for the first time and within about a week it became routine. Our outside dog was now an inside lap dog. He still savored hanging around outside, especially when Lucy or I had outdoor projects, but he was just as content indoors, especially on my lap.

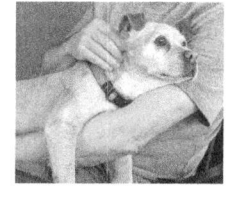

We had become nearly inseparable pals, and I had fully become "a dog person."

Seizures

Then, without warning, everything changed. In September 2019 Baxter had two consecutive major seizures that put him the ER for four days. He could not eat, drink, or move on his own. The doctors were preparing me for a discussion of euthanasia, and I was overwrought with grief unlike any I could have anticipated feeling for "just a dog."

But Baxter was not finished yet, and after four days, a healthy hospital bill, and enough tears to float a boat, he was amazingly able to come home. With mutual dedication to the task, we gradually rekindled all aspects of the life we had before the incident. Our walks around the pond took on new significance. I was ever so thankful to have been spared losing Baxter, an inevitability for which I was not yet ready.

Well, now he's gone and I'm still not ready. I know every day of the year and a half since his amazing recovery has been a bonus, but it's still too soon. And even as he gradually declined both physically and mentally, he continued to do all he could to please me until his last day. Hopefully he knew I endeavored to do the same for him.

Wake-up calls

I am grateful to have had the luxury of providing a peaceful exit for Baxter, resting comfortably and calmly on my lap without fear or pain, as the rain fell outside and the tears fell from my eyes and Lucy's.

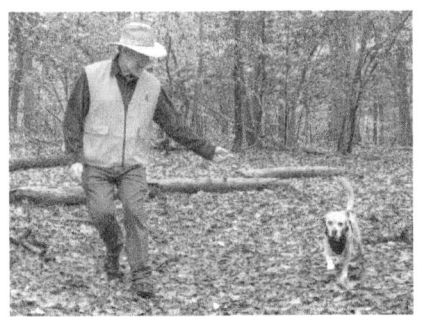

Today, a beautiful day full of sunshine, I received Baxter's ashes. So once again I put on my walking boots and my Tilley hat, and with his collar in my pocket and his ashes in hand, I embarked on our usual lengthy path through the woods and around the pond. I scattered Baxter's ashes all along the path where we spent so many memorable mornings. It will give me a warm feeling as I walk there without him, knowing that a bit of his physical presence remains.

So yes, now I am one of those people. I had sweet nicknames for Baxter, had acquired every creature comfort imaginable for him, spent a ridiculous amount of money on medical bills, and devoted an inordinate amount of time to ... just a dog. And I would do it again a thousand times over. I miss him every day, and I expect that even as the tears cease, the hole he left in my heart will remain.

I remind myself that the grief I feel from losing Baxter is proof of the joy he gave me for so many years. And now, knowing that a mere dog can give so much joy, I promise you that the phrase "just a dog" will never again enter my mind.

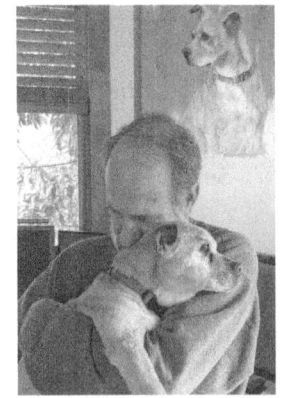

156

Just as prostate cancer was a wake-up call, losing Baxter was another. It seems we are destined to receive such wake-up calls periodically throughout life to remind us to pay attention. They are reminders to notice the good things, give them undivided attention, and love them. They will not be here forever, and neither will we. And although we know it is important to make the most of every day, it seems we need these wake-up calls to remind us to actually do it.

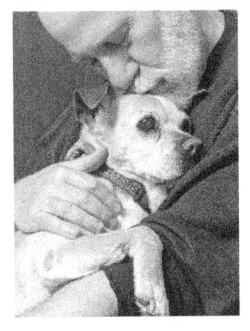

Thank you, Baxter, for all you taught me, and for all the joy you brought. You were one of a kind.

If you have a similar story, please share it with me. Thank you for letting me share mine with you, and for helping me honor Baxter.

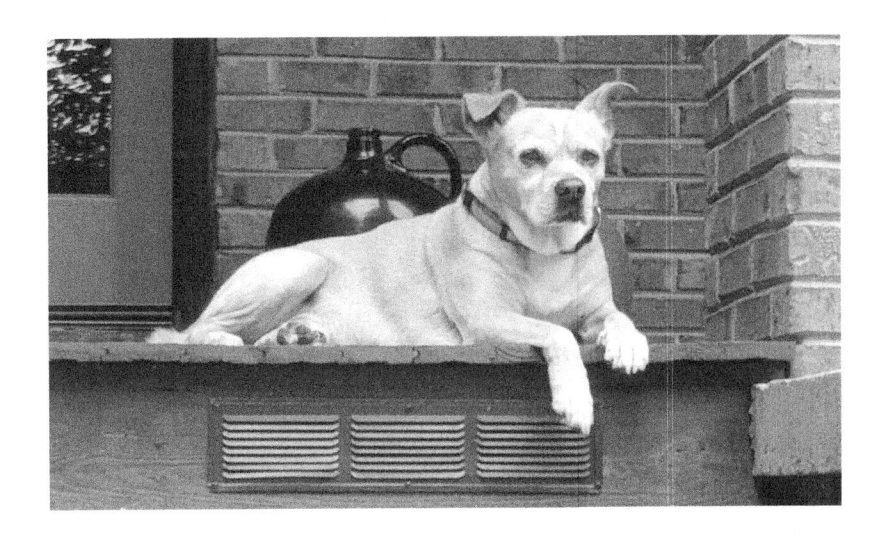

APPENDIX C:
The Stories Behind My Books

WHY MY FIRST BOOK?

In case you're curious, I would like to give you the inside story about why I wrote my first book, *PROTONS versus Prostate Cancer: EXPOSED* (2012). First, here's a super-short one-paragraph description for those who haven't read it.

Quick synopsis: Book#1, *PROTONS versus Prostate Cancer: EXPOSED*, is my detailed description of what it's like to receive proton beam therapy for prostate cancer. It's totally observational, non-technical, and very personal, told from the perspective of the patient (me). I did my best to leave nothing out, including the periods before, during, and after therapy. My goal was to provide ultimate detail about not only what was occurring around me and what was happening to me, but also what was going on inside my head and how I felt, so you could fully immerse yourself and make the journey with me. I hope you enjoyed the trip.

But why did I write it? Why bother? This is still one of the questions I am most frequently asked, and if I did not already know the answer, I would be asking myself the same question. After all, it was a major project, took a lot of my time for about a year, and I had no idea what I was doing in my first book-writing endeavor. I was a book-author-newbie.

I was also admittedly a self-confessed writer wannabe, but this is not why I wrote the book. For the record, here is the official Book#1 backstory of how and why it happened.

I was diagnosed for prostate cancer in 2010, treated in early 2011, wrote Book#1 during the remainder of that year, and published it in 2012. But I never intended to write it and had no foresight about doing so. I took no notes during my two months of treatment, other than jotting down the names of the wonderful radiation therapists ("RTs") who cared for me. I wanted to remember their names because more than anyone else, they are the ones who made the experience a positive one every day. To us patients, they were not nameless nobodies. They were very caring real people with names. They were *our* radiation therapists, and they became our most trusted friends for the duration.

On March 16, 2011 I completed my treatment and went back home to South Carolina, but the vivid memories lingered, continuing to roll around in my brain. And the more I thought about those two months, the more bizarre it all seemed. It was indeed a surreal experience.

On one level, I sometimes felt as if it were happening to someone else, while at the same time realizing the someone else was me. I suppose it might be akin to an out-of-body experience, which I've never actually had, so it's only a guess. You've seen those TV shows where the hospital patient, hooked up to a life-sustaining web of wires and tubes, lies on their bed as their ghost separates from them and floats above? Then the perspective changes to that of the floating ghost, gazing down at its body still on the bed, and after the spooky music stops, merges with the body becoming one again? Yeah. Like that.

This was how I watched myself experience proton therapy, and what I saw was not only extremely fascinating, but also seemed somehow important. Later, all those memories—from my urologist's shocking news, to the joy of rectal balloons, to making new friends, to the bittersweet departure upon completion of therapy—all of this mattered to me, and I feared that I'd soon forget the precious details. That would have been tragic, and for that reason alone I began compulsively writing everything I could remember, as quickly as possible, in full detail, just for me.

Every day after work I would spend hours at the computer typing random thoughts about every aspect of this once-in-a-lifetime experience, for no reason other than to remember it. Literally everything I could recall became part of this disorganized post-facto journal, written completely from memory without any notes. There was no structure to it, no coherent timeline, and no polish. There wasn't time for that because I was in a hurry to finish, fearful that I'd soon forget the detail. It was a massive, high-speed, frantic unfiltered brain dump.

As a side note, I'd already noticed that it is indeed common to forget much of the detail of what happened and how we felt, despite the vividness while it was happening, just as we quickly forget the details of a dream that was so clear and dramatic just minutes ago. Before I had decided on a course of action for treating my prostate cancer, I asked several former proton patients—proton alumni—to describe their experience. I'm a detail kind of guy, and I wanted all the details and quizzed them relentlessly. And although they were patient and willing, they were generally unable to provide more than general recollections. The forest, not the trees. I think this might be a male trait. We men live through it, and then we're done and move on. The big picture remains while the details fade.

I feared this would happen to me, and night after night I wrote, hoping to capture my memories before they faded. I was in my office at one end of the long hallway in our home, while Lucy was working in hers at the other end. After several months of this routine, Lucy, calling to me from the south end, asked me the question that changed everything:

"Hey, Ron! What the heck are you doing back there every night? Writing a book or something?"

Of course, Lucy didn't really suspect I was actually writing a book, and I wasn't. But by then I had indeed written quite a lot, and her question made me take stock and think about it differently. *Hmm, maybe it could be a book,* I thought. *Maybe all this inside-story detail would be useful to other men considering proton therapy. There's a lot of good information here. Why not organize what I've written and continue the story as if I were intending to write a book? If I become more intentional about it, maybe one day there might even be a book!*

At that moment I shifted gears. I was thereafter no longer recording randomly for my eyes only. I was purposefully producing a book to be seen by others. The closer I came to completion, the more necessary and urgent it felt to finish and share what I now see as a labor of love. It took me about a year, and the rest is history.

Okay, everything is history.

In hindsight, I am glad I wrote it. I am super-pleased that it has helped many people, some of whom made the effort to contact me for further discussion, to ask how I am doing, or just to say thank you. Even now, a decade later, people continue to find it useful.

I am indeed fortunate.

WHY ANOTHER BOOK?

Now you know that I had no plan to write my first book, at least not initially. Well, I can say the same about writing another, at least for many years after Book#1. For a long time I was quite adamant about not writing a second book because it made no sense to me to do so. Let me explain why.

Imagine that you are Neil Armstrong and have walked on the moon. First human to do so, at that. Pretty cool, huh? It's a once-in-a-lifetime experience that others will want to hear about, especially if they are considering a similar endeavor. They'll want details, so you write a book for them. Everything you can remember goes into the book. What happened to you before, during, and after the trip. What you did, how you felt, what you thought, saw, heard, smelled. Step-by-step from A to Z.

A lot of people read your book. They enjoyed and even benefited from your story. Inevitably, they started asking, "Hey, Neil! When are you going to write another book? I want more!" Well, great, you think to yourself, but you already told your walking-on-the-moon story in full, glorious detail in your first book. What can you possibly do for an encore? Walk on Mars? Go back to the Moon, taking an alternate route, or in a different kind of vehicle? Faster? Blindfolded? Backward?

The "write another book" question is a sincere and flattering request, so you politely respond with one of a few stock answers you've devised, like a simple and polite, "I currently have no plans for another, but you never know. Thank you for asking." Or maybe the slightly snarky and a tad sarcastic, "Hey, great idea! Never thought of that. Do you think I should? Maybe I will!" or "Soon! Soon! Be patient, I'm working on it ..." or "Funny you should ask, because I've already started writing one. It'll be my first cookbook—YAY—and if you liked my moon story, you're going to love my lasagna!"

Of course, few people want your cookbook or your pasta recipe. They thrilled to your space story and want more of "the moon thing," not a different thing. But as far as your moonwalking story is concerned, you've already told it. And you're probably not going to Mars anytime soon. Well, where does that leave us, eh, Neil?

Now, I am no Neil Armstrong, and nothing in my life comes close to his monumental accomplishment. But I did have my own once-in-a-lifetime experience, and like Neil, I wrote a detailed book about it. I am gratified that so many men and women have read my book and found it valuable. And I'm flattered that many of those readers have asked me if and when I would write another. And finally, the answer is …

Yes. Now.

Continuing the moon/lasagna analogy, I feel certain that my Book#1 readers were not hoping I'd write about my ongoing never-ending battle with the beavers who persist in eating my trees, damming my pond, and causing costly road washouts at the culvert they endeavor to obstruct. The once-in-a-lifetime experience I shared in Book#1 was a story of prostate cancer and proton therapy, not beavers. My readers would rightfully expect a second book to stick to the original subject, the one relevant to them.

But I've already told my story, and if a *Battling Beavers* book won't interest you, what am I to do? I admit to having felt at least a bit of "new book" temptation over these years, but I've been baffled about how to add to my moonwalk story. And the good people at the University of Florida Health Proton Therapy Institute refused to allow me to repeat my eight weeks there merely to gain new material for another book (apparently no double-dipping allowed). Having cancer is their typical minimum requirement, and I no longer qualify.

Nevertheless, after toying with the idea of writing another book for so long, I finally realize that now, ten years later, I do have a new and relevant story to tell. I have a decade of post-cancer life to describe. I've spoken with hundreds of men and women about their experience with this dreaded disease. I have seen the landscape of prostate cancer therapy evolve. And most importantly, I have learned a little about a lot of life.

I realized there is finally enough new stuff to fill a book. Might as well write it in case you want to read it. Hey, you *are* reading it, so thanks!

Well, truth be told, in my real-time moment today, I can only hope you will be able to someday read it because as I sit here now, still writing, I can't be 100% sure I'll finish my second book. For me, writing is tedious. I am not a fast reader or writer. Writing Book#1 took me a year, and my average rate of productivity was about 132 words per day, a lackluster performance for any serious writer. But I *am* serious, just slow. Okay, yes, and lazy. Plus, I procrastinate and perseverate. My motivation ebbs and flows, and I am easily distracted. Ugh.

With those undeniably counterproductive traits in mind, I will nevertheless push myself to reach the finish line. If I do get there, I hope you find the result to be worthwhile. After all, you are a dedicated reader of my writing. You could have skipped this chapter entirely, but you didn't, so thank you again for sticking with me.

If you're a member of the prostate cancer club, or the more exclusive proton subset, or maybe the much larger any-kind-of-cancer club, or a caregiver of one of the above, or a medical professional working with any of these communities, this book is for you, from me. I hope it has helped you gain insight into what life is like for at least some of us cancer patients during the decade after proton, after cancer, and beyond.

THE COVER PHOTOS

The cover photo for this book is totally staged and posed. Unlike Book#1, this one was intentional, so the need for a photo was expected, discussed, debated, planned, and professionally done. With two books, I am now a bonafide book author rather than a one-trick pony, and I can justify a real photographer. Oh, yeah!

Fortunately, Rick Smoak, a good friend of mine, is indeed a professional photographer. He graciously agreed to photograph me as the "new Ron" standing on the right side of this book's cover. I am in a very relaxed pose, pointing at the "old Ron" stolen from the cover of Book#1. I suppose I was sort of relaxed, if it's possible while someone (Rick) is softly, soothingly, but firmly providing a non-stop stream of instructions like *left foot an inch to the right, point a little higher, twist slightly toward me, stand up straight, suck in your tummy, chin up, push up your glasses, stand up straight, bigger smile, suck in your tummy, thumb in your pocket, suck in your tummy ...*

Thanks, Rick. It worked!

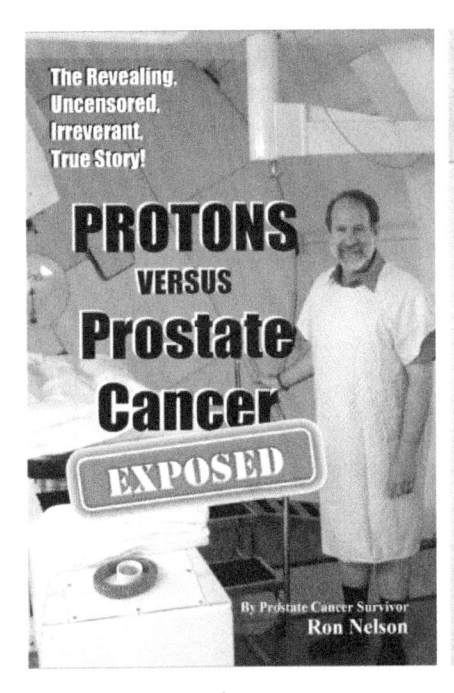

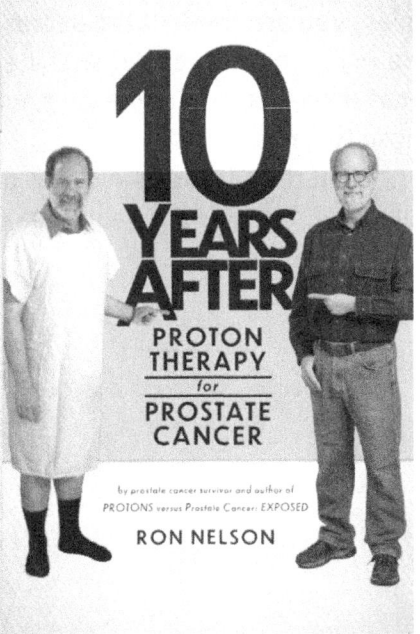

There was no professional photo for Book#1, my accidental book. I never even considered a professional book cover. Nor did I have any reason to expect to need a cover because I had no idea there would be a book, so during my proton therapy I did not take any noteworthy photos that might have become cover candidates. Frankly, I had other things on my mind. You know, like getting rid of my cancer and stuff like that.

You might then wonder, where did Book#1's cover photo come from. Did I revisit the gantry later, once there was a book, just to strike a pose?

Nope, I did not. The photo was taken by my daughter Jessica, who visited me in Jacksonville one weekend and asked if she could photograph me in my treatment room (the blue gantry), just for fun. As always, the RTs were accommodating and with a pretty good digital SLR camera, Jessica took what later became the cover photo.

But there was a potential problem. There were two RTs in the photo, and I knew using their images could have legal ramifications I preferred not to address. So, as an IT guy with some computer skills, I "photoshopped" them out, and you'll never know who they were unless you are them. It is a secret I'll take with me to the grave, just like my grandmother did with her previously mentioned recipe for what she called porcupine balls, which I remember fondly, along with those two RTs.

Here is Jessica's original photo with two of my favorite RTs still there, but unidentifiably cloaked in gray:

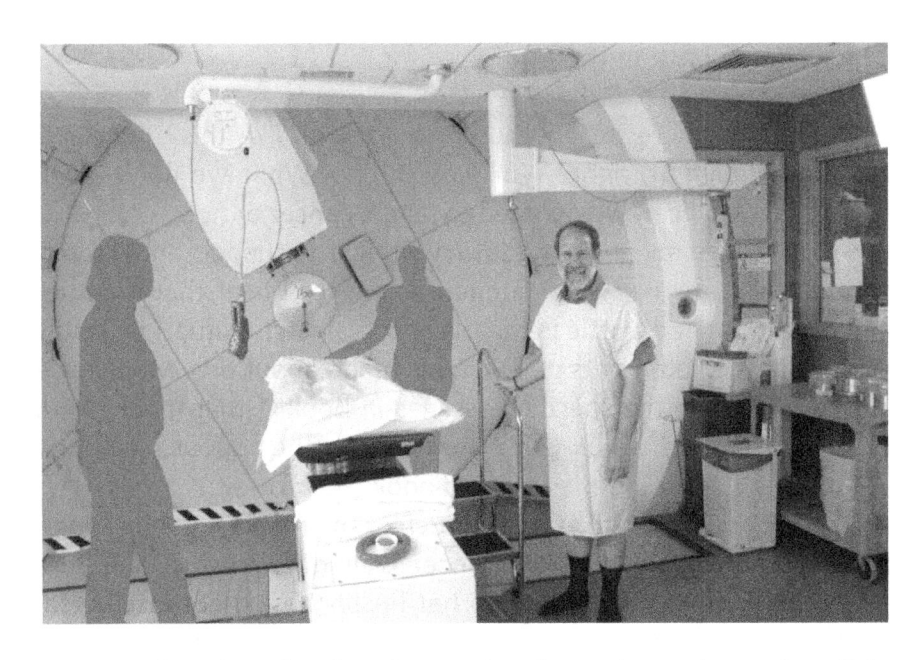

Other than the ghostly RTs, the photo shows the reality of the moment, stylish black socks and all. The open-back robe makes a wonderful fashion statement, and I am sometimes asked to don a similar gown to help people verify my identity. Apparently, I'm not especially recognizable without it.

Clark Kent is anonymous without his red cape, as I apparently am, sans polka dot robe.

THE HUMOR

Should there be any humor in a book like this? Cancer is nothing to laugh at, right? Well, yes and no. While we don't laugh about having cancer, we do need to laugh, cancer or not.

Although my primary goal in writing is to support and inform, not entertain, my day is brightened whenever I hear that a reader smiled and laughed a little in the midst of a stressful situation. I truly appreciate the comments people have made about this. Many have even pointed out the specific passages in Book#1 that made them laugh and told me which parts they read to their spouse. My first effort turned out to be a read-aloud book. Who knew.

And to my initial surprise, much of the reading aloud is done by women. Although prostate cancer is uniquely for us men, it is frequently the wife who reads to her husband, and not vice versa. Kudos to those women. Truth be told, we men do need a little help now and then, and maybe a gentle nudge.

After many years, I now have a pretty good idea how people have reacted to *Protons Exposed*, but your reaction to *10 Years After* remains to be seen. I sincerely hope you found a helpful thing or two here, and if it brought an occasional smile to your face, so much the better. If your load was lightened a little, it will make my day.

Suffice it to say that if I helped you see a serious matter from a lighter perspective in either of my books, I'm happy to have done so. After all, a little laughter or even a small smile is a big help after a bit of bad news. And while I don't believe laughter is the best medicine—I chose to be treated by a radiation oncologist, not a comedian—I do believe humor can ease the burden.

Fortunately, there was plenty to be found on my journey, and maybe yours, too.

> *Cancer is probably the most unfunny thing in the world, but I'm a comedienne, and even cancer couldn't stop me from seeing the humor in what I went through.* — Gilda Radner
>
> [Radner, G. (2009). *It's Always Something*. Simon & Schuster]

A SHAMELESS REQUEST

Forgive me. I am about to humbly ask you to consider submitting a review of this book. Shameless, I know, and I find it awkward to ask, especially because I know you are busy with pressing matters like, hmm, let's see, maybe fighting cancer?

But your review of either of my books will help people who have never heard of proton therapy find out about it. At the time of this writing, proton is still often omitted when treatment options are given to a patient, tragically leaving them ignorant of its existence. You can help fix this problem for future newbies who could benefit from the power of proton therapy, if only they knew about it. Your words will have an impact well worth a five-minute break from your cancer research.

Okay, here goes: If this book (or my first one) has been valuable to you in some way, I hope you'll take a few minutes to post your review. There. I've asked. It's official. That wasn't so hard, Ron, now was it.

Well, yes, it kind of was.

APPENDIX D: The Best of The After Proton Blog

After my first book was published and became a runaway hit (possibly a slight exaggeration), I have been frequently asked when I would write another. I allowed myself to feel flattered by what I'm certain was often little more than a conversational icebreaker rather than a serious request. Plus, I had my own doubts that a sequel would have been of much interest or use, even if I could manage to write one. I suppose you could call the book you are reading now an extremely belated sequel.

Still, about a year after publishing Book#1, I did have some new ideas. Not so much book-worthy, but thoughts worth sharing, nonetheless. My post-proton brain was still making observations beyond the final chapter of my book, and little by little the urge to share them increased. I had opinions, insights, inspirations, analyses, and reflections that needed an outlet.

That's why I created *The After Proton Blog*, an online home for my musings. Although I have a lot to say about practically everything, I generally restricted the subject matter of the blog to "perspectives on protons, prostates, and people ... from inside the mind of a prostate cancer survivor treated with proton beam therapy." Keeping within those boundaries, I have so far published about seventy articles dedicated to my past, present, and future proton brothers.

Some of my readers and good friends have suggested compiling *The After Proton Blog's* content into a book, but why bother? It's all online for free. Then again, books do have some advantages over blogs. For example, you can easily read a book in literally any room of the house. *Any* room. You can carry it with you to read without internet on a plane or a train, keep it on your nightstand, take it to the beach, or lend it to a friend. And a book will survive long after a blog withers on the web.

Still, for some reason the idea of *The After Proton Blog* in book form didn't sit well with me, and I am not sure exactly why. It might be because among those blog posts I have some favorites, as well as some I am not as fond of. Yes, that must be it. Okay, no book edition of *The After Proton Blog*.

But I do now have an opportunity to selectively share with you just a handful of the best of the blog as I see it, and that is exactly what I will do. Why not!

Consider this section a bonus freebee, no extra charge, stuffed between the book covers after its MSRP was already set. If your book seems to be bulging at the seams, this is why.

Without further ado, here are a few of my favorites in their original unedited form, with a new brief introduction to each.

Enjoy!

HANK'S HYPOTHESIS: POST-PROTON VERSUS POST-SURGERY

Many of my articles on *The After Proton Blog* are inspired by you. When you contact me to share your concerns and thoughts (please do!), you motivate me to ruminate, cogitate, and develop those ideas further. "Hank's Hypothesis" is a perfect example of this. It is a direct result of a specific conversation with one of you (not actually "Hank"), and is apparently something many others have contemplated, too. It surprised me by becoming one of the most popular articles on the blog.

I suppose it shouldn't have surprised me. After all, it is no secret that you and I pay close attention to our PSA. Some of us obsess over it, and others just keep a calm, watchful eye on it. The PSA level is an important number, often our first clue about the presence of prostate cancer. Later, once treated, it provides us with continuing reassurance that our cancer is gone. In the minority of cases, it warns us of cancer's possible return.

It is entirely feasible that by the time you read this the PSA test may have become obsolete, supplanted by a more consistently accurate or 100% definitive test. Regardless, the following blog post from 2017 will still apply by substituting the name of the new test for PSA. You'll see that the article is not about the PSA test, but rather our obsession with monitoring our status, particularly post-treatment.

Hank's Hypothesis:
Post-Proton versus Post-Surgery
April 10, 2017

A friend of mine—a prostate cancer survivor and proton patient I'll refer to as Hank—called me to discuss some comments he was about to post on a cancer forum. His premise was that although proton therapy for prostate cancer has many potential advantages over radical surgery, there may be one overlooked disadvantage he thought he should perhaps share on the forum.

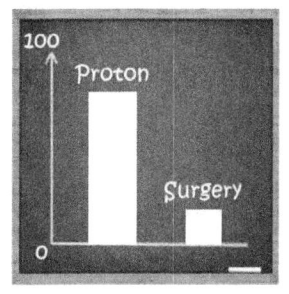

For the moment, I'll let you ponder what the alleged drawback might be.

173

I suspect other men in our prostate/proton alumni shoes have had similar thoughts to his. This is admittedly not an entirely new topic, but a subtly different twist on a familiar one. Before I divulge more about Hank's theory, we should briefly review the path that brought us here, for those who might not know. If you do, you can skip the next section with impunity.

Why we chose proton

Rarely is the option of proton beam therapy (PBT) handed to us on a silver platter. Surgery, brachytherapy, conventional radiotherapy, and other options are commonly offered as treatments worth pursuing. Sadly, it usually requires a patient's own proactive independent research to discover the option of proton. I and many readers of this blog took that initiative.

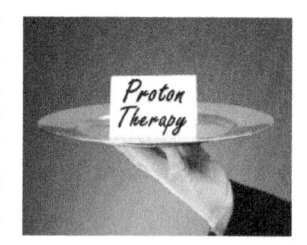

One way or another, we discovered non-invasive, painless, precise proton therapy and learned about its unique characteristics resulting from the Bragg Peak. Then we addressed the same inevitable, invariable questions we applied to all other alternatives: Will it cure my cancer? What is the likelihood of unpleasant side effects? Is it available to me, and can I afford it?

Cost and convenience aside (both improving in recent years), those of us who chose proton therapy for prostate cancer strongly believed it gave us the best chance to cure our cancer with no adverse side effects. We wanted to live a long, normal life, and were willing to fight for whichever treatment offered the most promise for achieving our goal. While we certainly understood that any therapy, including PBT, could fail or cause side effects, we believed— as most of us still do—that proton therapy was more likely than alternatives to leave us cancer-free without incontinence, urinary urgency, bowel urgency, or erectile dysfunction.

But we didn't consider whether it would leave us worry-free.

Why they chose surgery

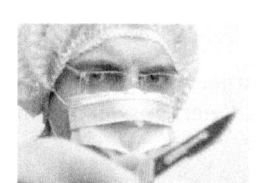

For some men with prostate cancer, there is a visceral need to "get it out," and surgery is the only way to satisfy their need. In addition, they may have heard surgery confidently referred to as the "gold standard" for curing prostate cancer. Whether accurate or not, who are we to say whether in their case, surgery wasn't actually their best bet?

They may have any number of other reasons for their choice to go under the knife. But it doesn't really matter. At the end of the day, every choice is highly personal, and none of us should feel the need to justify our choice of treatment to anyone but ourselves. We must live with the choice we made.

Regardless of how we proton patients may feel about surgery, we wish those who chose it no less than a complete cure with no side effects, and I'm sure this feeling is reciprocated. We are all in the same boat. They, like us, are seeking a return to their normal life. They, like us, chose what they believed to be the best path to achieve it.

And they, like us, didn't consider whether it would leave them worry-free.

Worrisome watching forever

After completing our treatment, we are not done. Whether we had surgery or proton therapy, we must watch our PSA—possibly forever—for the same two reasons. We know there was some chance the treatment might have failed to "get it all." We are also aware it can return if just a few undetected prostate cancer cells were hiding anywhere in our body—even beyond the prostate. As my ever-clever oncologist describes it, we can't always know before therapy whether the horse may have already left the barn. This is our reality, regardless of which treatment we chose.

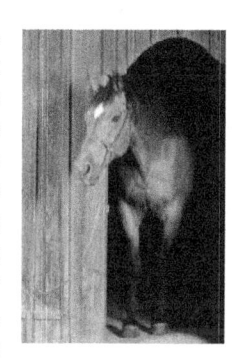

Not surprisingly, after treatment some proton patients worry. Some surgery patients do, too. We have all learned and have become hyper-aware that cancer can happen, even to us. We know if it happened once, it can happen again. We know there can be a new cancer, or a recurrence of the old one. With this awareness, can any of us ever return to our worry-free lives?

Who wins the worry war?

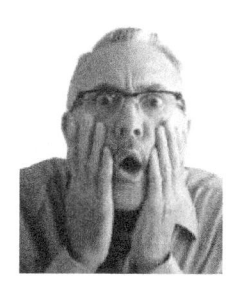

Men who opted for a radical prostatectomy expect a stable PSA of zero. After all, the prostate is gone. This means that for the surgery patient, very tiny increases can be worrisome. The James Buchanan Brady Urological Institute said this:

> The return of PSA is a possibility that strikes terror in the heart of every radical prostatectomy patient; in

fact, for many men, the dreaded follow-up PSA tests after surgery are almost worse than having the operation itself. What will you do if your PSA is no longer undetectable?

Would a similar assertion apply to proton patients? We who chose proton cannot expect zero. Instead, we eventually reach a nadir—our lowest PSA level—close to, but greater than zero. We'll still have a measurable PSA because with radiation, some healthy prostate tissue capable of producing PSA may survive the treatment.

We've been forewarned that our PSA might even jump around a bit. Maybe a lot. We know some increases are probably fine, and could be caused by a urinary infection, prostatitis, an agitated prostate, healthy prostate tissue, or various reasons other than cancer. We also know larger and/or consecutive increases could mean trouble. Does this possibility "strike terror in the heart" of every proton patient?

Surgery. Proton. For both, our post-treatment PSA is important. We watch it to make sure we're still okay. And because of its serious nature, we might worry about it.

But Hank wonders who worries more? Surgery survivors, or proton alumni?

Hank's hypothesis (at last)

I know it's unscientific to state the hypothesis near the end, but this is a blog, not a study. So here now is Hank's hypothesis. As he was feeling anxious about his upcoming post-proton PSA test, Hank found himself suspecting this:

> *Surgery patients have the post-treatment luxury of not needing to worry as much as proton patients.*

After all, Hank said, their prostate is gone and their PSA doesn't bounce around. Their PSA tests, he said, are generally routine, unremarkable line items in their lab reports. Although we proton patients know our PSA will not be zero and can jump around, even a tiny upward PSA movement can ignite a fear of failure or recurrence. We find ourselves facing a lifetime of anxiety surgery patients avoid, Hank postulated.

For the reasons stated above, this distinction seems unlikely. The PSA level remains a concern for all prostate cancer survivors, regardless of treatment modality. At least in part, I suspect Hank's hypothesis might have been a way of expressing his understandable envy of a stable PSA of zero, which is arguably a simpler state of affairs than his. But my guess is, if Hank had chosen surgery—or any alternative—instead of proton, he would still worry about every PSA test as much as he does now. We'll never know.

The bell curve of worry

I suspect the classic bell curve applies to our propensity to worry, more than to the treatment modality. I know of no formal comparative study of this, so it is an educated guess. It seems likely that at one end of the bell curve we'll find a relatively small group of men capable of nearly complete compartmentalization of PSA worries. They may feel a little anxious just prior to each test, but between tests they rarely give it a passing thought. At the other end of the curve are the men who worry daily, and sometimes work themselves into an emotional frenzy as each test approaches.

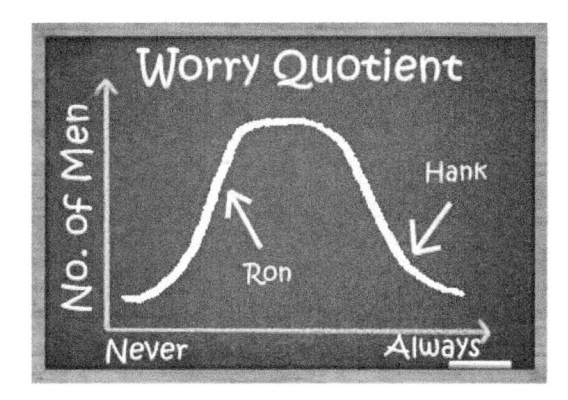

Each extreme is a minority. Most of us are in the middle hump of the curve. We have some level of constant awareness and concern, but manage it well enough and live a largely normal life. However, Hank might find himself closer to the worrisome end of the bell curve. Hank is a worrier, and he would not be doing less of it had he chosen surgery instead of proton. He would be just as anxious about every PSA test.

Non-discriminatory worry

Hank's hypothesis might have seemed reasonable at first, but after discussing it with him, he ultimately agreed it is not. It is not only flawed, but also unfair to both surgery and proton patients. Surgery patients are by no means exempt from post-treatment PSA anxiety, and proton patients are no more likely to be anxious.

A quick perusal of the many online prostate cancer patient forums will corroborate this view. Surgery, proton, or whatever—we all watch our PSA for the reasons stated above. Read the forums and you'll find an abundance of commiseration, concern, compassion, and relief about PSA levels from any prostate cancer survivor treated in any manner. There are no dividing lines relating to treatment modality.

Let's thank Hank

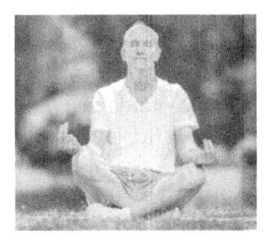

I'd like to thank Hank for inspiring me to think about this. It won't make me worry more or less than I do now, but it will remove any suspicion that surgery would have resulted in a more worry-free existence for me. I'm somewhere just left of the middle of the bell curve, and there I shall remain.

Should you be more worried? Should you worry less? If you are a worrier like Hank, you'll worry. If not, you probably won't. Neither cancer nor how we treat it changes this personality trait. We are who we are.

Do you think surgery patients worry less than proton patients? Where are you on the bell curve of worry?

SOUP, COFFEE, AND CANCER TREATMENT

I am passionate about precision in language and frustrated by the frequent lack of it. Sometimes it matters a lot, while at other times it may be trivial. But who is to judge? Better to err on the side of truth and accuracy, which I endeavor to do. But it requires a commitment not everyone is willing or able to make.

As a recent example of the importance of this, the unfortunate plight of my son-in-law who has MCAS (mast cell activation syndrome) is perfect. I'll leave it to you to research this disease, but the bottom line is simple: if he eats the wrong food he can have an immediate and fatal allergic reaction. He must therefore be vigilant about consuming only safe spices, oils, and literally every component of any recipe you can imagine. If he asks whether the meal you are serving contains a particular seasoning, it is a most serious question needing a precise, truthful, accurate answer, which is often hard to come by.

My earliest lesson in language precision was provided in my high school math class where Mrs. Pankin, a personal hero in my education, would not tolerate imprecision. She would ask us to provide instructions for drawing a square, and with chalk in hand, would follow the given directions exactly as stated. The initial naïve instruction to "draw four lines" evolved into "draw four lines of equal length" to "four connected lines of equal length," and eventually to "a quadrilateral with four equal sides and four equal angles." It was entertaining, enlightening, and exhausting. And I loved it.

Along with her, Mrs. Citron, my beloved English teacher, would not allow needless vaguery, and literally banned the use of words like "get" and "interesting" in our writing assignments. She rightly claimed that such words had multiple alternatives providing more precise meaning with greater specificity (e.g., does "get" mean receive? become? obtain? feel? etc.) I confess to still using those forbidden words on occasion, but not without a twinge of guilt and the expectation of points off.

Now, more than a half-century later, I listen and hear what people say, knowing it might not necessarily be what they mean. I have learned to make a greater effort to glean their intended meaning, remaining aware that it is not always the literal one. Often, as in casual conversation, the distinction is of little consequence, but at other times precise communication can be crucial.

Shirley Citron might be pleased to know that I tackled this issue in *The After Proton Blog*. If you know where she is, I hope you will send her a copy of my article. But please, Mrs. Citron: no points off.

Soup, Coffee, and Cancer Treatment
December 11, 2017

Remember when we could ask a question and have a reasonable expectation of a truthful, clear, direct and to-the- point answer? I'm not sure I do. We Americans seem to have boxed ourselves into a prison of vaguery, avoidance, and circumvention. There is no one else to blame—we did this to ourselves, intentionally or not, and now we are paying the price.

We have made it horrendously difficult to distill the precisely pertinent information we seek about nearly anything. This certainly applies to our health, but first I'd like to illustrate why we find ourselves in this predicament by means of a simple analogy: soup.

Is there meat in that soup?

My wife likes soup, but doesn't generally like any kind of meat in it. At home this is no problem, but the restaurant scenario is different. We see a delicious-sounding soup on the menu, and Lucy will ask our server—let's call him Skip—a seemingly simple question:

Is there meat in that soup?

This is the simplest of questions. It's unambiguous, and there are only two possible answers—or so it would seem. But Skip finds a third reply, "I don't think so." Now, what are we to do with this information? Trust Skip's instinct? We asked because it's important to Lucy, so we continue with, "Are you sure?" to which Skip predictably replies, "Pretty sure."

Skip's motivation

Why does he respond this way? We might presume Skip to be merely lazy. His answer might be a disguised version of "I don't know, I don't care, and

I'm not going to offer to find out for you." But let's give Skip the benefit of a doubt. Maybe he's actually making an educated guess. He might know that their chef rarely uses meat in soup, translates this into "probably not," and innocently fails to realize we don't want to play the odds—we want a definitive answer.

Or maybe he does know there's no meat, but is afraid to tell us. After all, what if for the first time there is meat? It's certainly conceivable. What if he tells us there is none, and then it turns out he's wrong? What if Lucy is allergic to meat? What if she becomes deathly ill? There could be dire consequences for Skip—risks he is reluctant to accept.

In defense of Skip

Sadly, he would be justified because as a society, we have made Skip's nightmare scenario plausible: He tells us there's no meat, but there is meat, Lucy gets sick, we sue Skip and the restaurant, and Skip becomes jobless, possibly bankrupt, and maybe unemployable. You know it could happen this way and so does Skip, so he behaves accordingly. In fact, noncommittal answers have become automatic for him. This behavior has become part of his deeply embedded internal survival programming. If we're serious enough about wanting the soup, we could ask Skip to check with the kitchen staff and find out for sure. Armed with a definitive answer from the chef—the only person who knows 100% for sure—Skip can now safely convey to us an accurate one-word answer, acting as merely the chef's messenger..

Without gaining access to the chef, Lucy would have to gamble based on inconclusive information. What we have here is a lack of resources— there's only Skip. And he is not a good information source because of the fearful environment we've created. We're stuck.

Is coffee good for me?

The story of Skip and the soup illustrates one end of a continuum. Now let's look at the other end: an abundance of resources and too much information. Instead of soup, let's consider the often maligned and equally revered beverage that's near and dear to my heart: coffee. The question is again simple:

Is coffee good or bad for me?

I suppose I could go back to the restaurant and ask Skip, but I have many, many other resources for coffee. And if I'm serious about changing my behavior based on the answer, I'll make the most of all available resources. Once again, I need one of those elusive single-syllable answers. So where do I begin?

Coffee: ask the experts

In no particular order, I'll start with my ENT, who is now fully vested with me, having examined my ears, nose, and throat. The latter has given me some trouble lately, which seems to be related to reflux, which is apparently worsened by (among other things) coffee. Dr. ENT says, "No more coffee," and without hesitation I say, "Nice theory, doc. Not gonna happen." He also said to drink fewer colas, and with that I'll comply, so I feel vindicated.

In any case, another of my many highly regarded doctors recently listed coffee consumption as a way to greatly minimize or reduce the risk of prostate cancer onset or recurrence. Music to my ears! Even better, to have this benefit I apparently must drink at least four cups daily. Excellent! I am now adhering to at least one doctor's advice.

Two doctors: one says "bad," the other says "good." So far, it's a tie.

But I really do want an answer. To break the tie, I do some online research. Shooting for the bullseye, I google "is coffee good or bad for me?" There are over a quarter billion results for that question. Well, I'm retired and have time to tackle the list. Here are today's first four results:

    12 Health Benefits and 6 Disadvantages of Coffee

    Coffee and health: What does the research say? – Mayo Clinic

    Coffee: Good or Bad? – Healthline

    Is Coffee Good For You? Is Coffee Bad For You? | Time

To be sure, the main benefit of coffee for me is simple: I like it. I find that it relaxes me and gives me great pleasure. Until it is shown to have an indisputable dire consequence similar to that of smoking cigarettes, I will continue to drink it—probably four or more cups a day.

Bottom line: I now know a lot more (but not everything) about how coffee could be helpful or harmful to my health, and I still don't know whether I should drink it. But I do.

How should I treat my cancer?

It might seem like quite a leap from soup and coffee to cancer, but with a cancer diagnosis we must confront the same fundamental issue. The consequences are more significant, but the challenge is the same. How do we find the right answer to an important, unavoidable question? In this case, it might be phrased like this:

    Which of the *available* cancer therapies is best for me?

This is not a yes-no, good-bad question. It is multiple choice of tremendous complexity. Regardless, with a cancer diagnosis or recurrence, choosing an answer is unavoidable. And when it's our question, we can't help feeling that it somehow must be answerable.

Cancer: ask the experts

So we ask our urologist, who happens to be Skip's brother, Dr. Kantsay. He gives us our list of options. We are pleased to know there are choices, and now we want him to tell us the right one. But like his brother, he won't commit for much the same reasons. What if he's wrong?

Kantsay might tell us which therapies other patients have been happy with. He could even indicate his support for whatever decision we make. But he's not going to put his neck on the legal chopping block and pick one, even if he privately feels certain about which is best. We'd like him to ask his team of experts in the kitchen—radiologists, physicists, oncologists, urologists, dosimetrists—and then relay their answer. But this is life or death, not soup, and even the team won't commit.

We decide to seek a second opinion, hoping for a definitive answer—and we get one. We see Dr. Kutter, who turns out to be a distant cousin of Kantsay. Dr. Kutter is likewise a urologist, as well as a surgeon specializing in performing radical prostatectomies. He explains why surgery is the gold standard for treating prostate cancer, and doesn't hesitate to recommend it. While Kutter sounds convincing, the bias is not hard to spot, and we are left no further ahead.

In fairness to the doctors

To be fair to Dr. Kutter and others like him, we must not equate their bias with their motive. They may sincerely believe that surgery—or whatever the bias may be—is the gold standard, and best for us. Of course, some may have ulterior motives, but I suspect they are the exception.

To be fair to Dr. Kantsay and our many unbiased doctors, we must allow the possibility that even the best of them might not have the answer we need. They're not necessarily withholding information out of fear; they just don't know. They are in the same boat we are.

Worse yet, some questions have no clear answer. And others have several legitimate, but differing answers. Dr. Kantsay might not be able to give us our answer because there is none, or there are too many. Either way, we're not going to like it, and will undoubtedly move on to the next step.

Cancer on the Internet

We've spoken to Kantsay. We've heard from Kutter. Now we're on our own, and it's up to us and Google. With keywords "best prostate cancer treatment" we are rewarded with over a million results. Feeling a little pressed for time, we try to only consider credible sources.

We are surprised to discover additional options that were not on the original list provided by Dr. Kantsay. We find that combinations of therapies are also options. Our research is leaving us even more confused and torn.

Like coffee, we quickly discover that even credible sources disagree on which cancer therapies are good or bad, let alone which is best for me. We research and read until we're weary, and find ourselves again knowing a lot more than we did, but still lacking the ultimate answer. Yet, we must decide.

Between a rock and a hard place

In trivial matters and serious ones, we often find ourselves stuck between too much information and too little guidance. We find plausible-sounding justification and support for diametrically opposed conclusions. We encounter objective experts who are understandably afraid to commit or just don't know, and biased ones who sadly will, often with genuine conviction.

When we try to sort out the mess ourselves, we drown in a sea of data, statistics, and opinions that offer justification for virtually any position we ultimately decide to take. Finally, we might even have to accept the infuriating reality that either we'll never know which answer was right, or that the right answer is currently unknown, or even unknowable.

Nevertheless, life goes on and for better or worse, we must make decisions. Soup, coffee, or cancer therapy—it's up to us. Sometimes we'll be wrong, sometimes we'll be right, and sometimes we'll never know. Such is life.

So do the best you can. Take your pick, make your choice, don't look back, and have a happy new year! And keep in touch!

DISCLAIMER: Skip, Dr. Kantsay, and Dr. Kutter are fictitious. If you happen to know anyone with those or similar names, rest assured my characters are not them. If you know anyone with different names but similar attitudes or behavior, I won't be surprised.

PROSTATE CANCER AND THE CHEESECAKE FACTORY

Soup, coffee, and now ... cheesecake? If you think I'm obsessed with food, you're not entirely wrong. It's probably the reason it occurred to me to compare bias in restaurants to bias in medicine. It is a fun way to make my point, which I described and referenced in various parts of this book.

The point is this: there is a lot of sometimes annoying but perfectly reasonable bias everywhere, which can work to your advantage if you recognize it for what it is and understand why it exists.

Let's have a little fun with this concept by comparing the bias at The Cheesecake Factory with what we encounter in our medical community. And while you're reading, why not enjoy a tasty slice of your favorite cheesecake along with a hot cup of the best coffee you can find.

Prostate Cancer and
The Cheesecake Factory
March 6, 2020

With the fast-growing number of options for treating prostate cancer, our decision about which to choose has become increasingly difficult. In the old old old days when it was surgery or a likely premature death, the limited list of options made the choice a little clearer. Unless there was good reason to expect a quick departure from this world for reasons other than cancer, I suppose we'd probably find a good surgeon with a sharp scalpel and hope for the best.

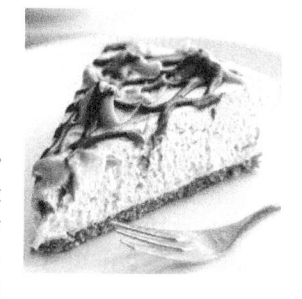

Nowadays our prospects are bright, but we must make a much more complex choice between conventional surgery, robotic surgery, cryosurgery, x-ray/photon radiation (IMRT), brachytherapy, hormone therapy, chemotherapy, gene therapy, HIFU, and (my personal favorite) proton therapy, to name just a few. We must also consider various intensities, frequencies, and combinations of the above, further increasing the number of line items before us.

It's as daunting as making a selection from the 19-page menu at The Cheesecake Factory.

Choices abound. How in the world can we make sense of it all and make a good decision? It's tough, and everyone will want to offer their two cents worth. And whether curing our cancer or our hunger, the influencers operate in surprisingly similar fashion. Our challenge is to understand and remember the motives behind all this well-intentioned advice so we can keep it in the proper perspective.

Let's consider three areas of influence you'll encounter as a customer at The Cheesecake Factory or as a prostate cancer newbie.

The server's favorite

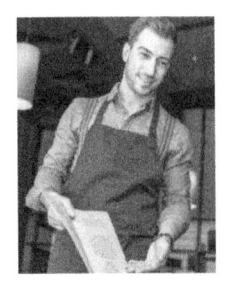

You walk into The Cheesecake Factory (TCF). The server welcomes you and delivers their massive menu, possibly in a wheelbarrow. After some serious perusal of the options, you decide to go with the Bistro Shrimp Pasta from page 8. Your server then excitedly declares, "Wow! Good choice! That's my favorite dish!" Similarly, a more aggressive server might initially hand you the menu, turn to page 8, point, tap three times, and proudly proclaim, "This one's my personal favorite. You should try it!"

This happens to me quite often, and each time my unspoken reaction is, "Well, hey, that's cool, but why should your favorite matter to me?" My favorite flavors might be entirely different than the server's. I might even be allergic to shrimp. Is there any reason to think the server's reasons for preferring the Bistro Shrimp Pasta apply to me at all? Unless I had asked for an opinion, the unsolicited comment seems totally subjective and irrelevant.

In the prostate cancer world, the urologist is often the one who presents the menu of treatment options, and you should not be surprised if you detect a not-so-subtle server-like bias. "My personal preference," you might be told, "is surgery. It's the gold standard. If I were you, it would be my choice. I highly recommend it."

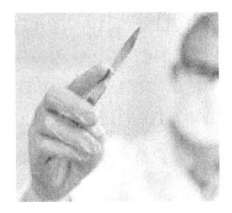

Regardless of the urologist's reason for this preference—and urologists are certainly entitled to have one—it is just one person's opinion. And although your request for the doctor's professional opinion is implicit, the prudent response is to research and explore the other options thoroughly on your own. Surgery might indeed be the right choice for you, but you can't know this until you've given the rest of the menu equal consideration.

There are as many flavors of prostate cancer therapy as cheesecake, and you will eventually develop your own very personal reasons for preferring one over the others. Once you do, run with it and don't look back.

The chef's recommendation

Talk to any chef at The Cheesecake Factory and you'll probably find that they also have a personal favorite dish, but for different reasons than the server. The chef not only knows how good their concoction tastes, but also takes pride in the skill required to prepare it properly. They might favor a recipe they invented, or one they are supremely qualified to execute.

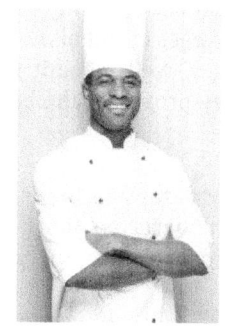

At TCF, the chef who prepares the dish is unlikely to also be the server who presents the menu. But with prostate cancer, the urologist is often both the server and possibly your chef, not only providing the list of treatments, but also speaking as your potential surgeon. This dual role can make the urologist's influence even more intense, doubling the force of their guidance.

Indeed, many if not most urologists are surgeons trained in conventional or robotic surgery. They naturally and rightfully believe in what they do, and there's nothing wrong with that. It is understandably their favorite because they've invested considerable time and money in learning how to do it, but that doesn't mean you must necessarily share their viewpoint. You can appreciate the enthusiasm, acknowledge the skill, and then choose to agree or disagree.

One chef at TCF might believe their Pasta Da Vinci (page 8) creation is simply to die for, and will recommend it at every opportunity. A skilled surgeon might sincerely believe daVinci robotic surgery is the gold standard for prostate cancer treatment. Both are respectable views worth hearing, provided we consider the source and keep them in the proper perspective.

The house special

It's not hard to guess what The Cheesecake Factory is most famous for. Indeed, two full pages in the menu are devoted to variations of their signature delicacy. Once I've finished my meal, should I be surprised to hear the server ask if I'd like to try a slice of cheesecake?

Likewise, and happily so, medical facilities have specialties, sometimes proudly represented in their name. My treatment alma mater, the University of Florida Health Proton Therapy Institute (UFHPTI) makes no secret of their specialty, even though they can also provide (for example) conventional radiation when appropriate. Nevertheless, their main attraction—the house specialty—is unquestionably proton beam therapy, and they are especially proud to be one of its earliest pioneers.

While the staff of the Cheesecake Factory will be happy to tell you about their Lemoncello Cream Torte if you ask, their enthusiasm for cheesecake will predictably be greater. Likewise, the staff of a proton center will be most eager to trumpet the unique benefits of proton beam therapy, even if they offer other treatment options, too.

There is a justifiable bias associated with having a house specialty in any field, and it's not a bad thing. If we remember to expect it and allow TCF and UFHPTI to describe their respective specialties, we'll benefit from their experience and the first-hand information they provide. Who better to tell us about cheesecake nuances than

TCF? The same applies to surgery hospitals, brachytherapy facilities, and cancer treatment centers of all flavors. Let them describe the house specialty, such as it is. Then make your own informed, very personal decision.

It's all good

Today's menu for treating prostate cancer is as amazing and extensive as that of The Cheesecake Factory. Choices abound, and the already high likelihood of achieving a successful outcome is still on the rise. But choosing a path is increasingly challenging, and it's not easy to exert a consistent effort to sift through all the well-intentioned advice. Easy or not, we must be aware of predictable biases and make the necessary effort to see the entire cancer therapy landscape clearly and objectively.

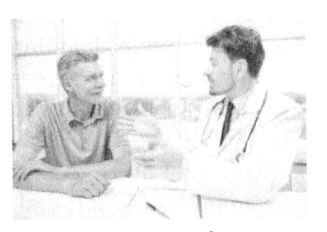

So choose wisely, and enjoy your cheesecake.

I'm curious: was proton on your menu?

5 REASONS PROTON PATIENTS ARE SO DOGGONE HAPPY

Did you read the earlier section called "A private conversation with proton ambassadors?" Of course, unless you are one, you were not expected to read that section. Regardless, consider yourself exonerated if you can recall the phenomenon I referred to as *proton euphoria*. I first noticed this in 2018 and was inspired to write about it then, years before I coined the phrase.

Indeed, proton patients do seem unusually happy, and in this article I enumerated some reasons why. Put them all together, add a little sugar and spice, stir a bit, and wahlah! Proton euphoria!

While I am no longer euphoric, ten years later I am absolutely still happy. Today it seems quite fitting to reiterate and summarize some of the reasons why, which conveniently happens to be what I did in my 2018 blog post.

If you are a prostate cancer newbie, I want to paint the picture of a future full of happiness for you, too.

May you find happiness in every remaining day of your life.

---

5 Reasons Proton Patients Are So Doggone Happy
April 22, 2018

At the end of this post I'll discuss the important exceptions that make the rule. What rule? We proton patients are a happy bunch—maybe even happier than the rest of the general population. This is a non-scientific personal observation based on more than seven years of being a prostate cancer proton patient.

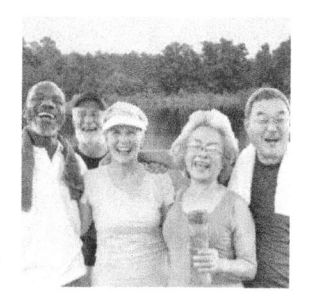

The notion occurred to me after a recent trip to my treatment alma mater, the University of Florida Health Proton Therapy Institute in Jacksonville. I visit UF Proton several times a year to dine with patients at their Wednesday lunches, to speak at their prostate cancer clinics, and for my own annual checkups.

Jacksonville is a five-hour drive, and as a devout homebody and recluse I am loathe to leave home for any reason. So why repeatedly make the trip?

At this point it's completely optional and routine because thankfully, I'm doing fine. And although I certainly enjoy the company of my Florida oncologist, my friendly local urologist—just a 30- minute drive—is perfectly capable of effectively executing my annual DRE.

Happy people

So why make the trip? The answer is simple, if not obvious: I like being around happy, upbeat people, and I find them in abundance at UF Proton.

On the surface, this makes no sense. After all, this facility is populated by patients who without exception have had some very bad news. Who in their right mind can be happy about a cancer diagnosis? I wasn't, and I'm 100% sure that's universal.

Then how, under such seemingly dire circumstances, can we be so happy? I have a little insight by virtue of many conversations with others in my shoes. And there's also the guy who is literally in my shoes. So I'll speak for myself, and you can let me know if I'm also speaking for you.

Introspection

I am a member of this group, and a happy guy. This was also true before my cancer diagnosis. Cancer is not the reason I'm happy, but it has undeniably changed my perspective on life.

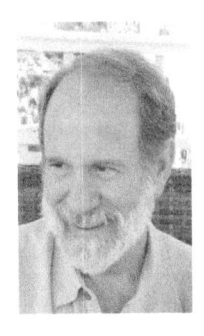

I have become more aware of the many things to be happy about. This may sound a bit trite, but it is the crux of the matter.

Before cancer I was happy enough, but not particularly focused on that feeling. I was just living my life, day by day, without paying much attention to the big picture. Now, with a recalibrated perspective I am laser-focused on the grander scheme of life. This has not only made me happier, but also more aware of being happy.

Let me tell you why.

Reason #1: I appreciate life more

"You have prostate cancer." Yikes. Was he talking to me? At that moment, at age 60, I instantly understood—I mean really understood—I could die tomorrow. Or today. Furthermore, I became acutely aware that I not only could, but surely would. This was not new information, but only then did I fully comprehend it.

I also quickly realized I still had no idea whether cancer or something else would eventually cause my inevitable demise, but the new insight lingered. From that day forward there would be a lot less lumbering through life. Without knowing it, I could be in the path of a runaway bus just around the corner, any time, any day. Best to take nothing for granted.

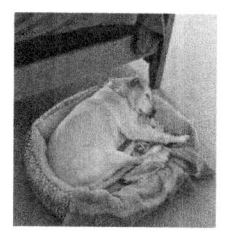

So how does this make me happy? With this insight comes a newly enhanced daily pleasure. I begin and end each day in a comfortable bed with the love of my life at my side, and my loyal canine companion at my feet. I am hyper-aware of their timelines as well as mine, and smile each morning at the sight of them.

This brings me a peaceful contentedness and makes me happy.

We cancer patients have become intensely aware that as a resident of planet earth, our timeline is finite and of unknown length. Everyone surely knows this, but not everyone "gets it." Well, we do, and it changes us forever.

Reason #2: I discovered proton therapy

As is the case with many of us, the challenge of cancer turned me into a researcher. And like my proton brothers, I was lucky. I found out about a lesser-known, painless, non-invasive therapy offering a high probability of knocking out my prostate cancer without side effects. I discovered proton therapy.

It was not proton that made me happy. I understood it would not be the elusive magical silver bullet, and as with any therapy, there would be no guarantees. But the way it works made sense to me. So much so that even if years later I were to find myself battling prostate cancer again, I could at least feel confident I had given myself the best shot in the first battle.

Finding proton gave me hope, and even the expectation that I would be okay. Today, seven years later, that vision continues.

Reason #3: I enjoy a unique camaraderie

For most of my life I was a shy, asocial introvert. I wanted to have friends and be a part of a close-knit social group, but it just didn't come naturally. Instead, I became comfortable enough going socially solo.

In Jacksonville life was different, and the social playing field was more level. Regardless of our path to Jacksonville, we were all in the same boat. We were all at least a little bit scared, as well as thankful and hopeful.

We patients didn't really have to become friends because we naturally were. We understood each other as no one else could, and with that comes an automatic bond and a unique camaraderie.

It's a feeling I like, and it still makes me happy.

Reason #4: I have more friends

Ours is a strong, enduring bond. I have many more friends now than before cancer. It's partly because of this camaraderie, and it's also because I've admittedly become friendlier and somewhat more sociable. I've changed.

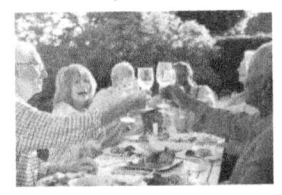

Some of my proton friends live nearby. In 2013—a couple of years after proton—my wife Lucy and I decided quite uncharacteristically to host a little party for local proton people. It was fun, and we have partied every year since.

In 2018, our fifth annual gathering, we had over forty proton guests from near and far. For some, it clearly required some time, effort, and planning to attend. I have asked myself why they made the effort, why many have returned year after year, and why our group of proton partiers has grown.

I believe the answer is this: we want to gather with others who understand us. And we like being around happy people. We miss the uplifting and inspiring companionship experienced during treatment, and this gathering is a chance for another taste of that, if just for a few hours. Our yearly get-together is not a support group, and it's not educational. It's just fun and revitalizing.

Reason #5: I don't sweat the small things

Size is relative. What once seemed large can quickly shrink when placed at the feet of the giant gorilla called cancer. And in an odd and slightly perverse way, I find myself in the gorilla's debt. It has forced me to focus my attention on the truly large things that really matter.

Many of life's little annoyances that drove me crazy before, now seem trivial by comparison. It's not that I don't notice them. I just don't care so much. A lukewarm meal that should have been served piping hot is just a lukewarm meal, not a life-threatening crisis. A favorite shirt ruined in the laundry by an ink pen I left in its pocket is a shirt I will remember fondly, not a reason to lose sleep. I have a long list of such things, and I'm sure you have your list, too.

So what matters to me now? If I were to tell you, it would sound preachy, so I won't. After all, my list is mine, as your list is yours. But since encountering the beast, my frame of reference has changed. Yours probably has, too, and it's for the better.

Our improved perspective of what's important in life should make us both happier people.

Happiness research

Perhaps surprisingly, research has shown that happiness is not about wealth or even health. It has more to do with realistic expectations and a positive mindset. Gratitude, exercise, meditation, and random acts of kindness contribute to our happiness. Greater tolerance of others, accepting that which we cannot control, and embracing our imperfect existence as human beings all bring contentment to our lives.

Most importantly, we have given ourselves permission to be happy now because we have grasped the uncertainty of the future. Contentment cannot be contingent upon our next PSA test, the stock market movement, or the weather. If we forever kick our happiness down the road in that manner, it will never be ours. And there is a lot to be happy about today.

The exceptions that make the rule

I acknowledge that some people are not happy, including some who have had neither cancer nor proton therapy. Everyone's life is a mixed bag, and any of us can easily find plenty to be unhappy about if that's our focus. I do know some proton patients who are doing quite well, yet are unhappy. I know others who face greater challenges and are nevertheless remarkably content.

What makes the difference? Clearly, our circumstances do not dictate how we feel. It's how we choose to respond to the hand we've been dealt that matters. We can choose to be happy, or not. Some fail to make that choice, while others try, but either can't or don't know how. In any case, it's not cancer, proton, or winning the lottery that will make us happy or not. It's our choice.

Proton brothers forever

Today I am clearly among the luckiest prostate cancer patients, but my circumstances could change tomorrow. Some of my friends—my proton brothers—have had a tougher time, battling a more advanced or aggressive prostate cancer, enduring multiple treatment modalities, side effects, or recurrence. Yet most of them still smile, laugh, and have a positive outlook.

That group could someday include me. I know it, and they know it. And regardless of our individual progress in battling the beast, we remain proton brothers. We continue to share a bond that cannot be broken, and appreciate each day in a manner unique to us.

Still, I ask myself whether I will continue to be happy when life gives me the next big kick in the pants. I say "when" and not "if" because it—whatever it will be—is inevitable. What if I have a recurrence, or develop some progressive, incurable neurological disease, or lose my eyesight? What if some Bernie Madoff drains my bank account? I like to think I'll still notice the remaining positive aspects of my life, focus on them, and find contentment.

None of us is pleased with the bad news part of the deal. But all of us in the fight can nonetheless be happy for much the same reasons.

We discovered proton therapy and found each other. We are riding atop the gorilla's head, and from there we have a new view of the world. We know what matters and have friends who share that view and understand us.

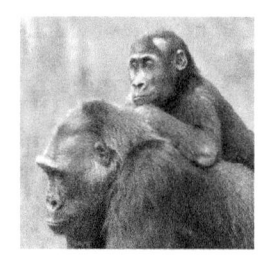

Such as it is, and in whatever quantity, life is good.

We can all be happy if we choose to be, so let's have some fun. Let's party.

QUIZ:

What do others say about happiness?

Here are a dozen quotes on that topic. Food for thought. See if you can guess who said what (I've included the answers). You will ace the quiz simply by reading the quotes, so relax and enjoy!

Also, please send me your own quote on happiness. Hearing from you will make me even happier.

QUIZ

Match these names to the following happiness quotes:

George R.R. Martin
Abraham Lincoln, Seneca
Paul Simon, Thomas Paine
Dalai Lama, Anne Frank
Oprah Winfrey, Buddha
John Lennon, Valerie Bertinelli
and Jerry Seinfeld

"Folks are usually about as happy as they make their minds up to be."

"Count your age by friends, not years. Count your life by smiles, not tears."
"Happiness is not something ready made. It comes from your own actions."
"Whoever is happy will make others happy."

"Laughter is poison to fear."

"Happiness is a choice. You can choose to be happy. There's going to be stress in life, but it's your choice whether you let it affect you or not."

"I've got nothing to do today but smile."

"I like money, but it's never been about the money."

"The real man smiles in trouble, gathers strength from distress, and grows brave by reflection."

"True happiness is to enjoy the present, without anxious dependence upon the future, not to amuse ourselves with either hopes or fears but to rest satisfied with what we have, which is sufficient ..."

"The greatest discovery of all time is that a person can change his future by merely changing his attitude."

"Happiness never decreases by being shared."

Answers are on the next page.
(no cheating!)

Congratulations! You have already passed this quiz just by reading the questions. And for clicking the answers button you earned extra credit, so you not only passed—you aced it!

Now send me your own quote on happiness (Ron@AfterProton.com). It can be your original words of wisdom, or something you've heard and want to share with me. Thanks!

QUIZ Answers

What do others say about happiness?

Abraham Lincoln:
"Folks are usually about as happy as they make their minds up to be."

John Lennon:
"Count your age by friends, not years. Count your life by smiles, not tears."

Dalai Lama XIV:
"Happiness is not something ready made. It comes from your own actions."

Ann Frank:
"Whoever is happy will make others happy."

George R.R. Martin:
"Laughter is poison to fear."

Valerie Bertinelli:
"Happiness is a choice. You can choose to be happy. There's going to be stress in life, but it's your choice whether you let it affect you or not."

Paul Simon:
"I've got nothing to do today but smile."

Jerry Seinfeld:
"I like money, but it's never been about the money."

Thomas Paine:
"The real man smiles in trouble, gathers strength from distress, and grows brave by reflection."

Seneca:
"True happiness is to enjoy the present, without anxious dependence upon the future, not to amuse ourselves with either hopes or fears but to rest satisfied with what we have, which is sufficient …"

Oprah Winfrey:
"The greatest discovery of all time is that a person can change his future by merely changing his attitude."

Buddha:
"Happiness never decreases by being shared."

MY COURAGEOUS BATTLE WITH COURAGE

Do you feel like a warrior fighting a courageous battle with cancer? I never did and still do not, but this is how many others characterize us. Just because I found myself in a minefield of risky alternatives does not make me courageous. Nor does it make me a victim, which is yet another common characterization I reject. I'm just a guy living a life full of challenges, including some unexpected ones, just like you and everyone else.

I must admit, I am not brave or courageous, although some will undoubtedly think I am simply because I was diagnosed with prostate cancer and seem to be "winning the battle." I just don't see it that way. Never have.

Looking back to my article of 2015, I see that I had to get this off my chest and confess. And I think I did a pretty good job explaining why I feel as I do, although I certainly respect your possibly different view. If you feel brave and courageous, and maybe you are, that is fine with me. Whatever the case may be, you are entitled and justified to see yourself as you do, and maybe as others do, too. In explaining my position, I do not mean to diminish or disrespect yours.

For the record, I still feel the same about this as I did in 2015, so here we go again.

My Courageous Battle with Courage
November 11, 2015

Since my prostate cancer diagnosis in 2010, my treatment in 2011, my 65th birthday last May, my retirement last June, and my upcoming death (no firm or projected date) I have been wondering what will be said about my demise when I'm gone. Hopefully somebody will say something, but what? I don't mean to be morbid, but I'd like to have some input about that.

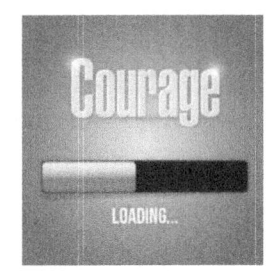

Describing my death

It will probably depend on how I die. I might drive off a winding mountain road in North Carolina and being Ron Nelson and not Bruce Willis, the tumbling descent would probably kill me. Or what if I just fell off a ladder and knocked my noggin on a rock? In either case there might be some reference to my tragic accident. Okay, that works for me.

When I was a single-digit kid I recall almost choking—the real kind: silent, scary suffocation—on a tiny bite of watermelon. What if a similar episode were to occur now, but without enough air in my tank to expel the tasty morsel across the room as I did then? Based on googling "choked to death" it seems choking inspires no adjective or judgment. I will have simply choked to death. Sad, but good enough.

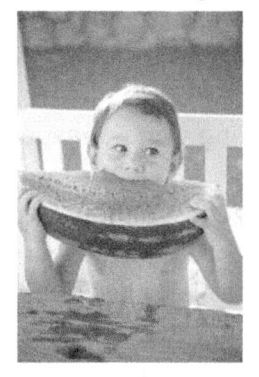

What if I shot myself while attempting to bag an 8-point buck or a belligerent beaver? What if the rifle was somehow defective or a ricochet followed an unfortunate path? In this case the focus of conversation would probably not be me at all. More likely, the story would be added to the stack of stuff promoting tighter gun control. I don't really relish becoming a posthumous political pawn, but I'd be gone and regardless of my personal views, that debate along with many other messy matters will be left to others. That's one of the few benefits of death, so I'll take it.

And what if I ultimately die of a prostate cancer recurrence or some other flavor of cancer? After whatever amount of time the available treatments buy me, what will be said then? We all know the likely answer:

Ron Nelson died after fighting a courageous battle with cancer.

Courageous? I'm really uncomfortable with that characterization, and here's why.

Courage and choice

Not only do I not feel courageous, by definition I simply do not qualify. Wikipedia's definition is as good as any:

> **Courage** *is the choice and willingness to confront*
> *agony, pain, danger, uncertainty or intimidation.*

The key word is choice. There was nothing voluntary about this—there was no sign-up sheet for cancer. After a brief but prudent period of biding my time (a.k.a., active surveillance) I did decide to treat it, but what was the alternative? If I die of cancer some may eventually refer to that period as part of my courageous battle with cancer, but please take note: I'm not brave or embattled. I'm just living my life such as it is, making necessary and sometimes difficult choices along the way.

The truly courageous

I particularly don't (and won't) deserve sharing the label of bravery with the many truly heroic men and women who chose an exceptionally dangerous, risky life to serve their country and mankind. Using the same adjective to describe me with respect to cancer is unfair to those genuinely courageous people I so deeply respect and appreciate.

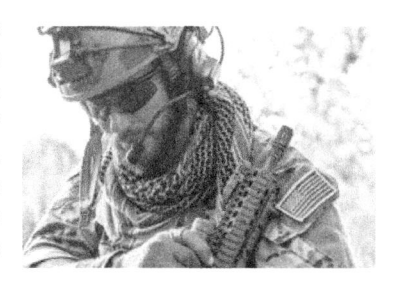

I did not fight in a war to serve my country as did many of my courageous proton brothers and others. The draft spared me (my Vietnam lottery number was a safe 364) and enlistment did not seem like the right path for me. I do not fly F/A-18 Hornets over Middle Eastern countries for the U.S. Navy as does my courageous son-in-law. I did not graduate from the police academy to serve my community in the face of daily danger as did my brave nephew.

Cancer was an unwelcome intrusion upon my life, plain and simple.

The scale of courage

There was no enlistment for my so-called battle with cancer. It was just a card dealt to me. I'm not battling or brave, and saying otherwise when I'm dead won't change the truth. I'm just living my life like you and everyone else with and without cancer.

In fact, so far I've had it pretty easy. I was diagnosed, treated, have no physical side effects worth mentioning, and can continue enjoying life. It doesn't get much better than that.

So if my death is ultimately from cancer, please keep some perspective about my realistic ranking on the scale of relative courage. I have no illusions about this and prefer not to be rated undeservedly high. This is not an effort to be humble, just accurate. Let's not dilute the genuine courage of those who actually deserve that label.

What research revealed

The Internet provided some interesting insight. I googled various keyword combinations to explore and test my assertion about courage. I searched for the phrase courageous battle combined with additional keywords including WW1, WW2, Iraq, Afghanistan, Vietnam, Korea, and others. The hit counts ranged from 13,600 (WW1) to 243,000 (Korea).

Then I combined cancer with courageous battle and there were a whopping 477,000 hits—more than double most of the others. Of course, these search results change constantly and this is not a scientific study, but it does indicate how the phrase is used—or misused—and I'm a little sad and disappointed by the result.

"courageous battle" cancer

About 477,000 results (0.34 seconds)

I am not alone in this feeling. During my research I stumbled upon the blog of a breast cancer survivor, Nancy Stordahl, who also wrote about courage and cancer. She effectively makes the point that words matter, and I couldn't agree more. In that regard, she says, "Let's not automatically turn to worn out clichés and war metaphors, even if well-intended." Thank you, Nancy.

Instinctive behavior is not bravery

Watching someone else undertake what appears to be a difficult or dangerous challenge inspires us to assign courageousness, but is it really? Behavior often looks like courage from the outside, but it's necessary to dig deeper.

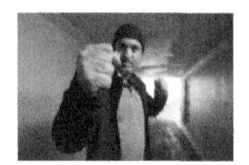

If I am mugged while walking in the park and react by trying to figure out how to fight or flee most effectively, would you think me brave? I did not choose to be mugged, but there you see me doing the best I can to prevail.

It would be accurate to say I was unlucky and victimized. It would make sense to say I was in the wrong place at the wrong time. You could certainly call me just plain unlucky at that moment. But merely doing what anyone automatically does in that situation would require no more courage than a non-swimmer gone overboard gasping for air. We would instinctively—not bravely—try to survive the ordeal.

And so it is with my cancer.

Life's risks and uncertainties

I know there could be a recurrence and confess to having a constant low level awareness of this unnerving possibility. Admittedly, it does take at least some effort to prevent that concern from becoming a more prominent fear. But other than doing some reasonable things to remain a healthy 65-year old hopefully paving the way to becoming a healthy 66-year old, there is not much to proactively do on a day to day basis. And merely living with concerns and fear does not make me brave.

What if there is ultimately another intrusion into my life by cancer or some other terrible disease? Will I then feel courageous for taking the next step to address it? This is only a guess, but I will probably just feel sad, angry and unlucky about it, will weigh the new set of risks served onto my table of life, and will choose the most acceptable combination.

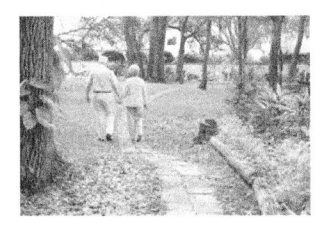

Cancer or not, we all engage in risk assessment every day. That's just life, not war, and not courageous.

Sorting it all out

Life is a journey requiring us to fight some battles, take some risks, and make some difficult decisions along the way. Courage is sometimes but not always required.

We should certainly praise and admire the strength and tenacity of those challenged by a serious illness. We should salute those who chose to bravely fight the important battles most of us cannot or will not fight.

And that's how I feel about being labeled as "courageous." What are your thoughts?

About the Author

Ron Nelson was born and raised in Michigan, graduated from the University of Michigan, moved to South Carolina soon afterward, lived in Charleston for almost twenty years, later moved to the rural midlands near Columbia, and does not play golf. He enjoys peace, quiet, solitude, birds, dogs and memories of Baxter, autumn, building fires, high octane fresh ground cold-brewed hot coffee, southern mustard-based barbecue, good movies and series, professional tennis, stimulating conversation, and many styles of music, especially finger-picking solo acoustic guitar.

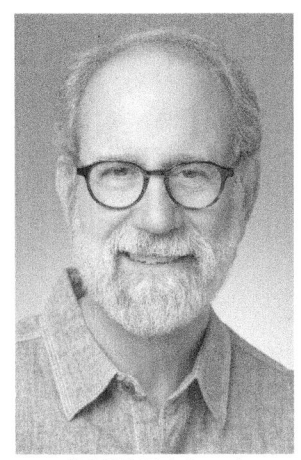

© 2022 Rick Smoak

Ron is the helplessly happy husband of Lucy, the proud father of four fantastic daughters (Julie, Jessica, Emily, and Caroline), four incredible sons-in-law (Brandon, Reed, Topher, and Mike), and the grandfather of eight terrific relatively new human beings (Dorsey, Ben, Anneliese, Joey, Henry, Max, Finn, and Ellen), so far. And he loves and admires his marvelous mother (Hecky).

Ron's careers were in music for ten years after college, and then in computers and technology until retiring in 2015. He is the author of *PROTONS versus Prostate Cancer: EXPOSED*, which details exactly what it is like to receive proton radiation therapy for prostate cancer, and he occasionally publishes his newest perspectives on people, protons, and prostates on *The After Proton Blog*.

Ron speaks publicly about prostate cancer and proton therapy when invited, and sometimes even when not.

Please contact Ron at **Ron@AfterProton.com**.
He'd love to hear your questions, comments, and stories.

Read more at *The After Proton Blog*
www.AfterProton.com

Now are you ready for the prequel?

PROTONS versus Prostate Cancer: EXPOSED

Time travel back to 2011 when Ron was treated with proton therapy for prostate cancer, and it was all new to him.

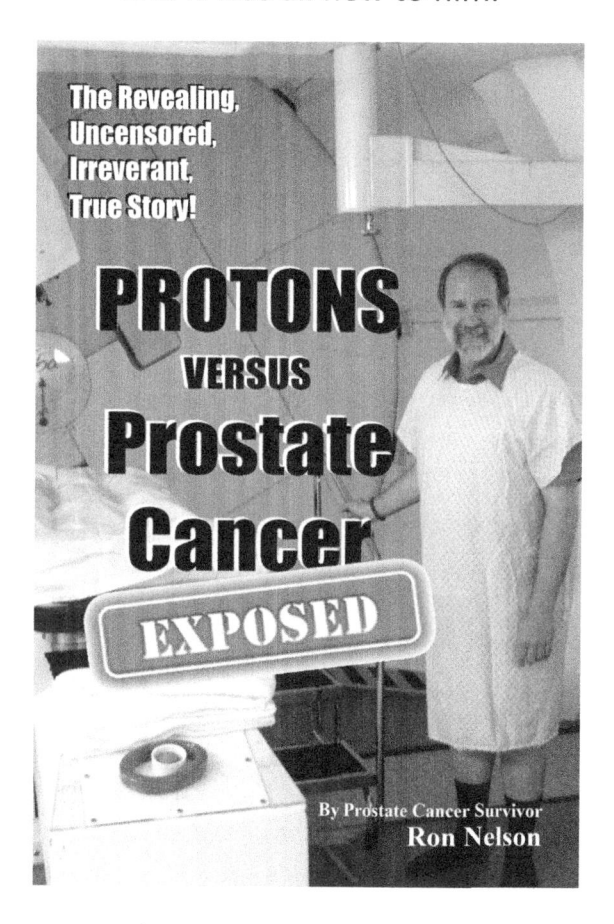

Experience the entire process exactly as he did, step by step, thought by thought, zap by zap.

Made in the USA
Middletown, DE
03 January 2024